Your Real
Superpower
Is Your
Body

World's **First Kid's**
Infotainment **Nutrition** Stories

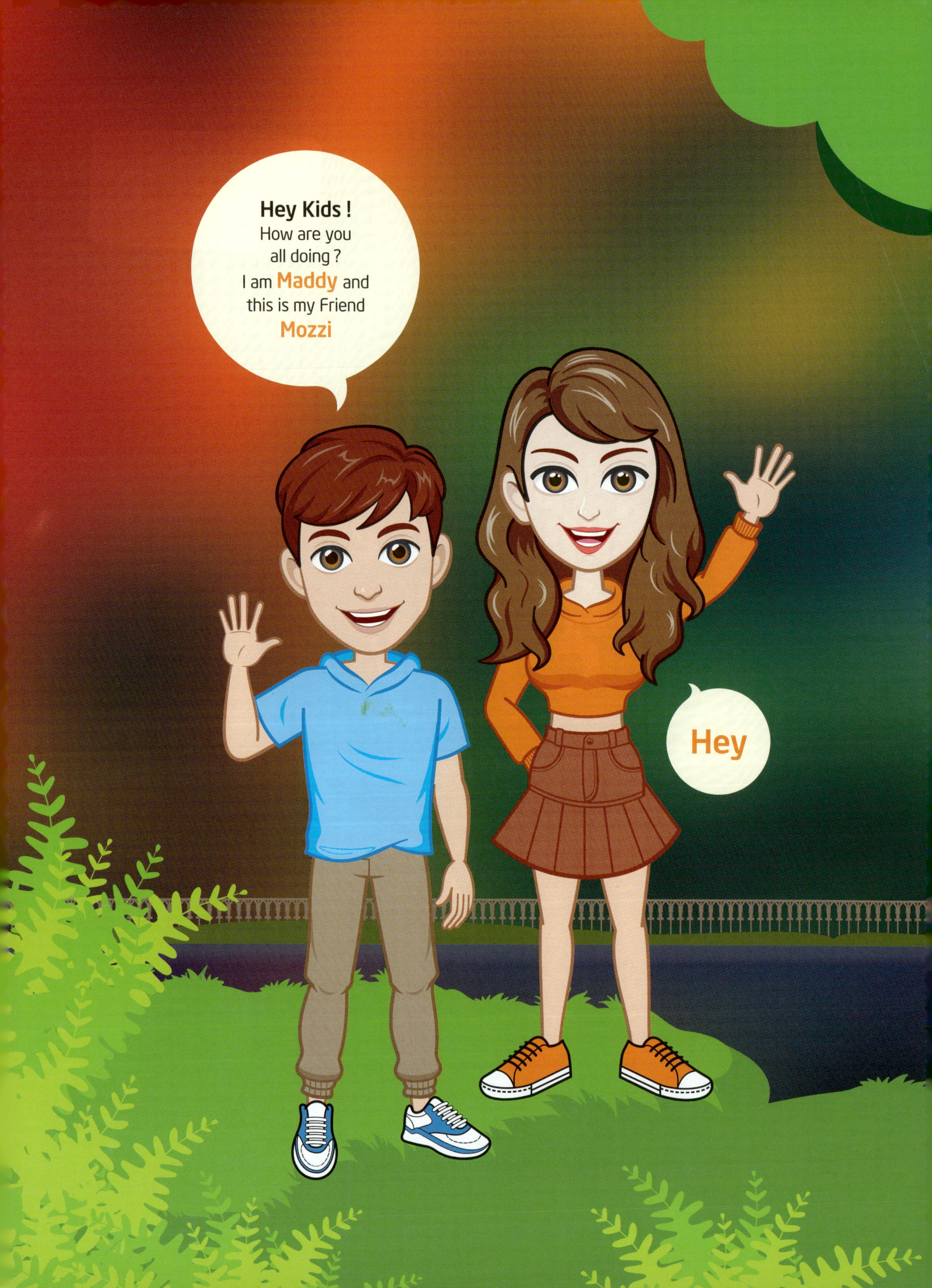

Hey Kids !
How are you all doing ?
I am Maddy and this is my Friend Mozzi
Hey

Greetings to all

It's not just what you eat, but your eating habits that define you and are important for a healthy lifestyle.

Kids these days take food without much thought, the only thing that matters to them is it's taste no matter how unhealthy it is.

For kids, everything they consume should satiate their taste buds. In today's time, with unhealthy food habits, most of the kids are suffering from obesity or are undernourished i.e. they are victims of malnutrition.

Good nutrition is a crucial symbol of our body status. To prevent losing it, one must not eat junk or unhealthy food, rather one should practice healthy eating habits.

We need to understand that there are always two sides to the coin.

The kids mostly consider food as complementary to entertainment. For instance, most of the kids eat junk food in theaters while watching movies or when they are stressed. They consume extra food or no food at all. We need to understand that food should not be based on need of time, but it should be based on the need of our body.

Few Important Notes for kids

- You are the base for your own body, In order to make yourself strong you have to follow basic principles of healthy lifestyle and diet.
- Your role in kitchen gardening –Try to make your own garden, plant some vegetables and fruits or plants of medicinal value.
- Your role in kitchen – Try to make some healthy dishes and think about what are the nutrients in your food.
- Your role while watching T.V. or movies – don't eat while watching a movie or T.V.
- Instead of wasting huge amount on junk food like Pizza, Burger, etc. try donating for a good cause to the needy. Many kids don't even get enough food to satisfy their hunger.
- Try to work out for at least 45 minutes daily and be active throughout the day.
- Apply all food groups and food plate system (NIN) in your everyday meal.

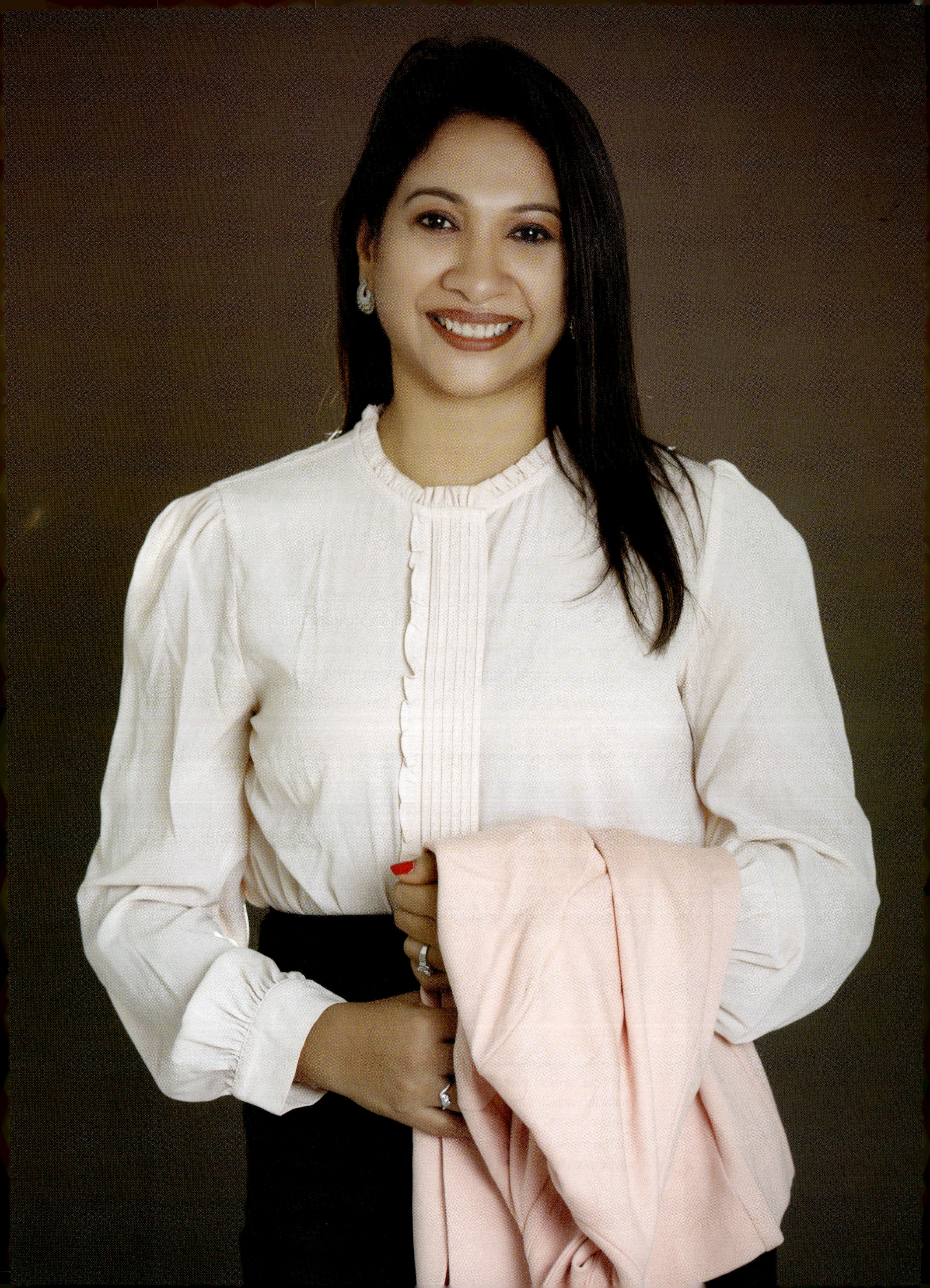

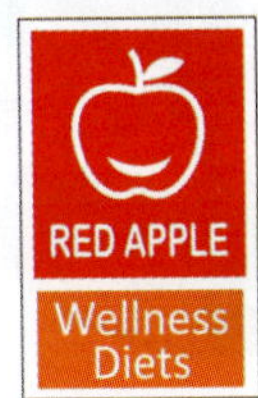

Meri Kalam Se

Writing a book is harder than I thought and more rewarding than I could have ever imagined. None of this would have been possible if this lockdown situation hadn't happen.

Due to a changing lifestyle & the environment around, there are many changes in food consumption patterns. Having an idea and turning it into a book is as hard as it sounds. The experience is both internally challenging and exciting. With my expertise in this field I found that new nutritional guidelines & requirements are arising on a day to day basis because of new research & development which has changed our vision and direction.

"Sowing seeds today & nurturing them will reap fruits tomorrow".

Keeping this idea in mind I am inspired to publish this book, as today there are very few books which help kids realise the value and importance of nutrition. In this book you will come across many engrossing & interesting facts for kids which will help them to understand how to apply them in their day to day activities.

With tremendous hard-work & efforts I have completed this book in 15 days.

Keeping a notepad & pen handy I hardly slept during this time. Whenever any idea popped up, I noted it down.

I hope you enjoy reading this book.

Dt. Meghana Kumare

Foreword By

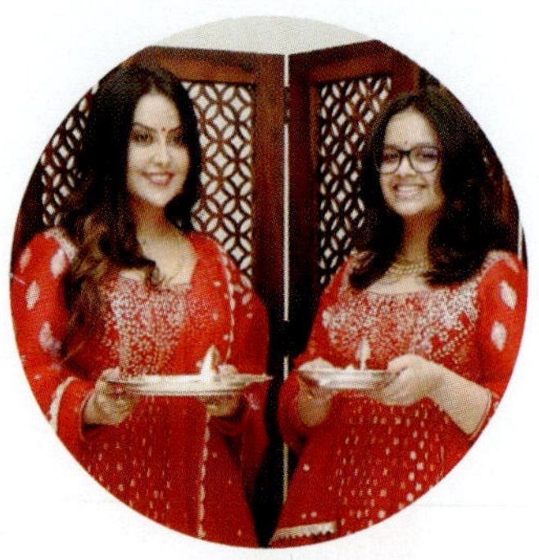

In Today's times unhealthy eating habits create greatest lifestyle problems in our lives. Fast food, Junk food-culture in our younger generation has caused increase in lifestyle diseases. Meghana has explained the concepts of nutritional values and food choices the youth has, through two characters namely Maddy and Mozzi in her book. It highlights common mistakes a youngster does, replacement food they can choose and active lifestyle they should maintain via regular exercise. The book will educate and encourage the youth to eat well and guide them on variety of foods which will help them to follow healthy and balanced diet. I feel that this is the kind of information which should reach every child so that they learn to take care of their physical health and develop healthy eating habits.

Best wishes for your book.

Amruta Fadnavis

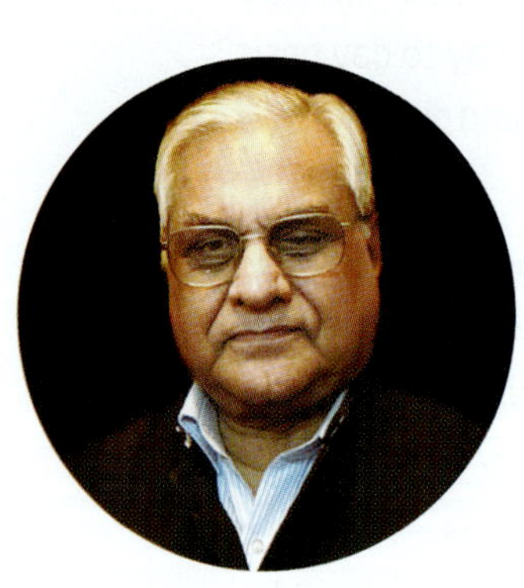

Dt. Meghna has very rightly tried to explain the basic reason of Malnutrition among kids that they mostly consider food as complimentary to entertainment . Reality is that right nutrition, from the Very begining can help in a child's growth and develop Healthy lifestyle habits. Making suru that children eat a balanced and nutritious combination of food is an essential part of their physical and mental development. Ensuring that a child gets the right nutrients is an important parental role. It is important to install healthy eating habits at an early age so that they can carry the habit with them as they transition through adolescence to adulthood.

In order to implement a healthy sustainable lifestyle, it is important to understand what good nutrition consists of . This book by Dr. Meghna provides great insights on nutritional knowledge. The specific breakdown of grains, proteins, Vegetables , fruits, nuts and dairy etc. , based on size, age and gender helps to decipher what does a balanced diet consist of. This will help both the parents and the children to understand food and nutrition as they grow older and also help to implement and maintain well balanced eating habits.

I visualize that Dt. Meghna's sincere efforts should reach the desired hands so that they may bear cherished fruits of her labour in transforming kids and moms into Superkids and Supermoms.

I wish her all success in this endeavour.

Ravi Dev Gupta
Chairman
Ekal Vidyalaya Foundation of India

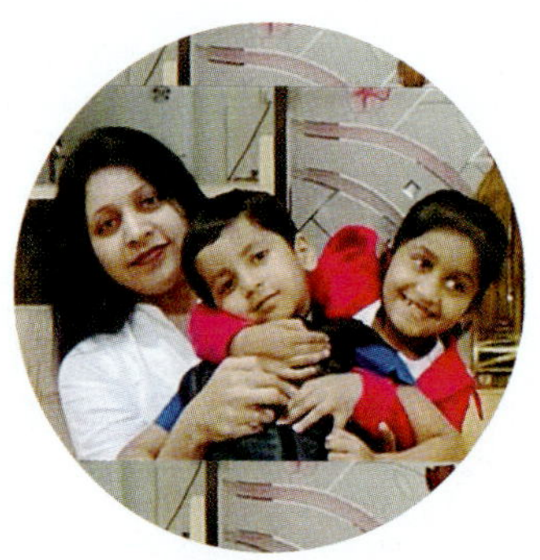

Nutritional values inculcated from the developing years of childhood creates healthy habits of mindful eating. There could be no better way to teach nutritional values to kids but through the superhero graphic stories, which is made so fascinating, attractive and informative by my dear friend Meghana in this book. Meghana's immense knowledge of diet carved out from the perspective of a child's interest plus psychology presented in the form of handy book is the greatest privilege of a kids and their parents too to sow the seeds of healthy habits.

Best wishes!

CA Shwetali Thakare
Member Economics Maharashtra Water Resources Regulatory
Authority Government of Maharashtra

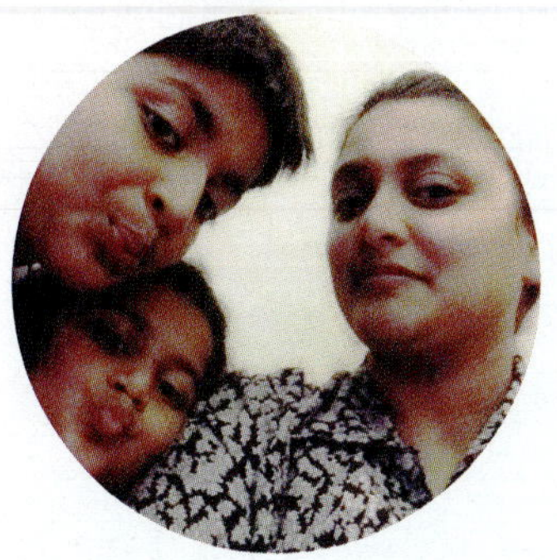

As any other parent I also wanted my kids to be happy n healthy. Happiness and kids are synonymous to each other but health n kids are not always the same.Kids love eating healthy or unhealthy, whatever they like and this was one of the major issue of worry for me.This book written by Meghana kumare attracts a child's attention as it has the portrayal of facts from the child's point of view hence they are interested in reading it.The comic characters add to the charm n knowledge of the children.This book is one of the best gift any parent can give to their children.

Best wishes!

Vrinda Meghe

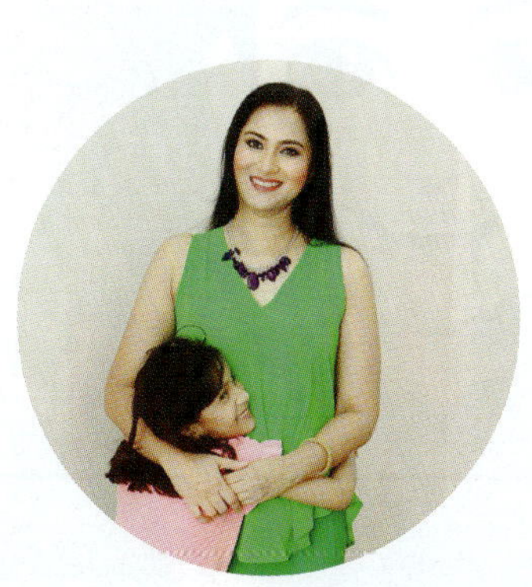

This nutritional book by Dt Meghana ji is a wonderful visual treat for kids and she has made it interesting by putting accross important nutritional suggestions via story tellingEarlier parents used to read and they used to implement it on kids . But this way the child is clueless as yo why he or she is being asked to eat a particular food .But this book is surely going to be pathbreaking as through stories the children will themselves understand what is the importance of healthy eating and will themselves make healthy choices rather than someone else forcing them for it .I congratulate dt Meghana ji for this brilliant informational book and making it interesting through her unique way of presentation. I'm sure the kids of all age groups will be highly benefitted from it.

Healthy kids .... Healthy youth ... bright future.

Dr Vartika Patil
MBBS MD MRCP Pathology
Director Dr Patil's Laboratory
CEO Founder Dr Vartika's Confidence Academy
Consultant Pathologist At Neuron Hospital
Mrs Universe West Asia
Mrs Universe Fabulous
Mrs Gladrags Top 10

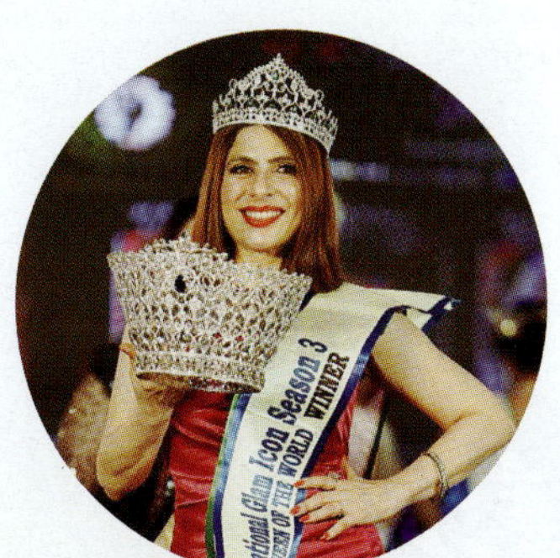

Meghana is a very intelligent dietitian who can give exact diet plan according to the persons requirements..and beleive me her diets really work..She has chosen such a great topic for her book as children are the futures of our nation ..and she's helping nation to become strong.. Congratulations dear Meghana for this wonderful book on a very apt topic.

My best wishes for your endeavour..

Vinita Bhatia
Fitness industry expert since 17 years Winner Mrs India
International glam 22 Mrs India beauty of World 22
Times of India "Most inspiring woman 22"
Times of india "Fitness Icon 22"

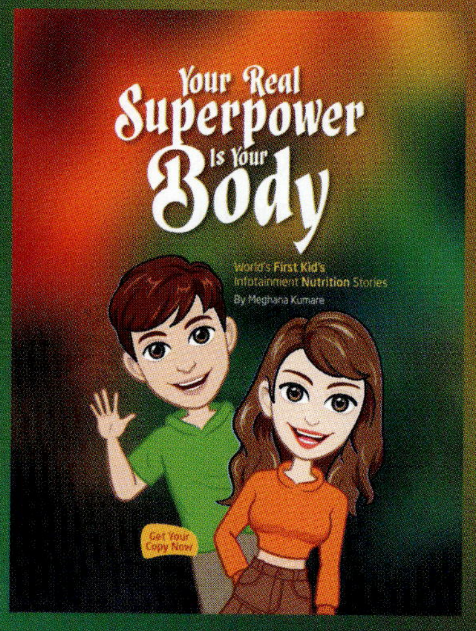

The Kid's health needs healthy eating plate, which is a guide to help, educate and encourage children to eat well and physical activities as part of the equation for staying fit & healthy.

Eating a variety of foods keeps kid's meals interesting. It's also the key to a healthy and balanced diet. The Kid's eating plate provides a blueprint to help parents make the best eating choices.

Author
Meghana Kumare

Illustration, Designing & Printing
Sanjeev Mendhe

Publisher
Dattsons Publishers

First Edition 2023

© Copyright reserved with Meghana Kumare

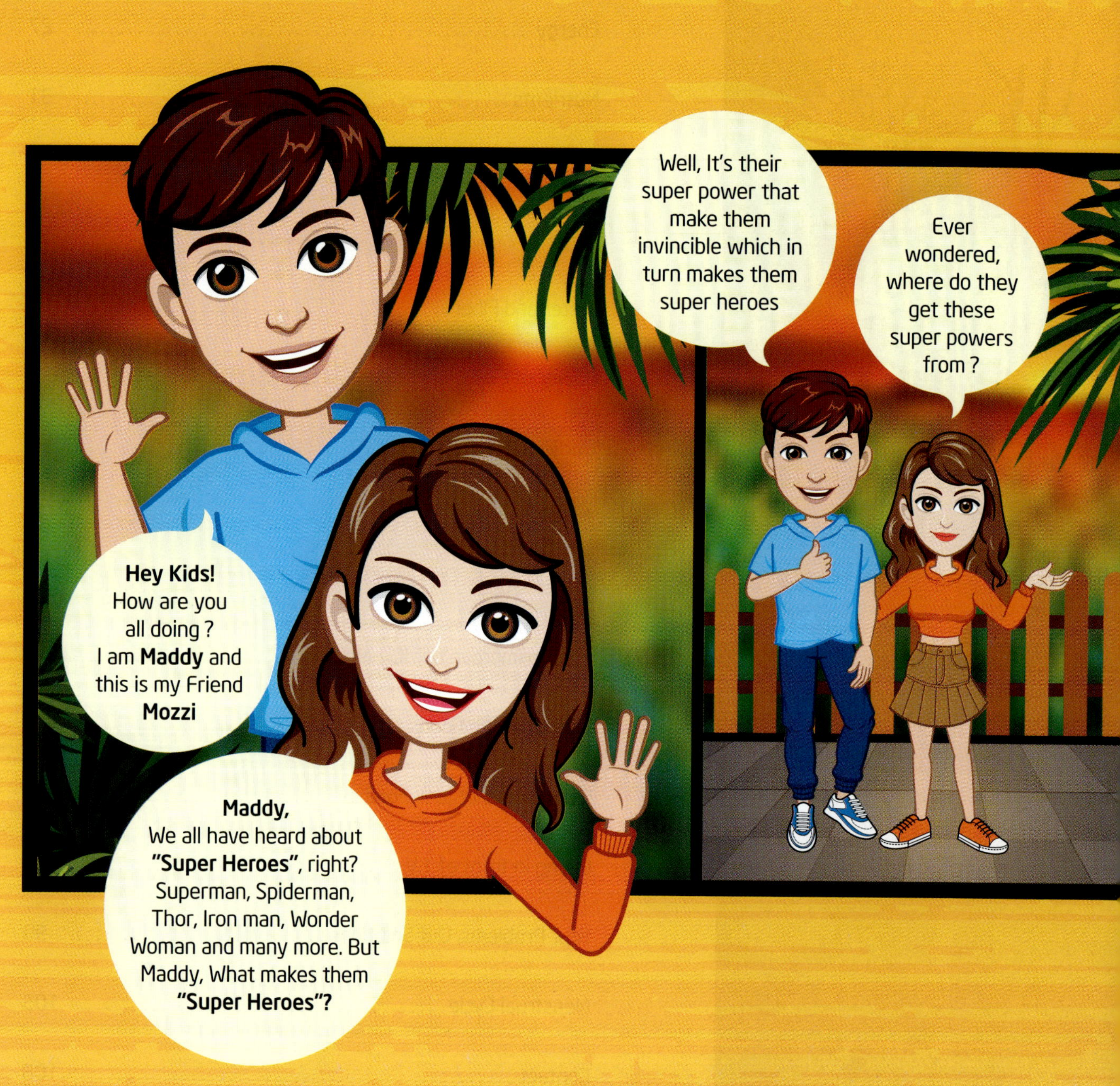

Hey Kids! How are you all doing ? I am Maddy and this is my Friend Mozzi
Maddy, We all have heard about "Super Heroes", right? Superman, Spiderman, Thor, Iron man, Wonder Woman and many more. But Maddy, What makes them "Super Heroes"?
Well, It's their super power that make them invincible which in turn makes them super heroes
Ever wondered, where do they get these super powers from ?

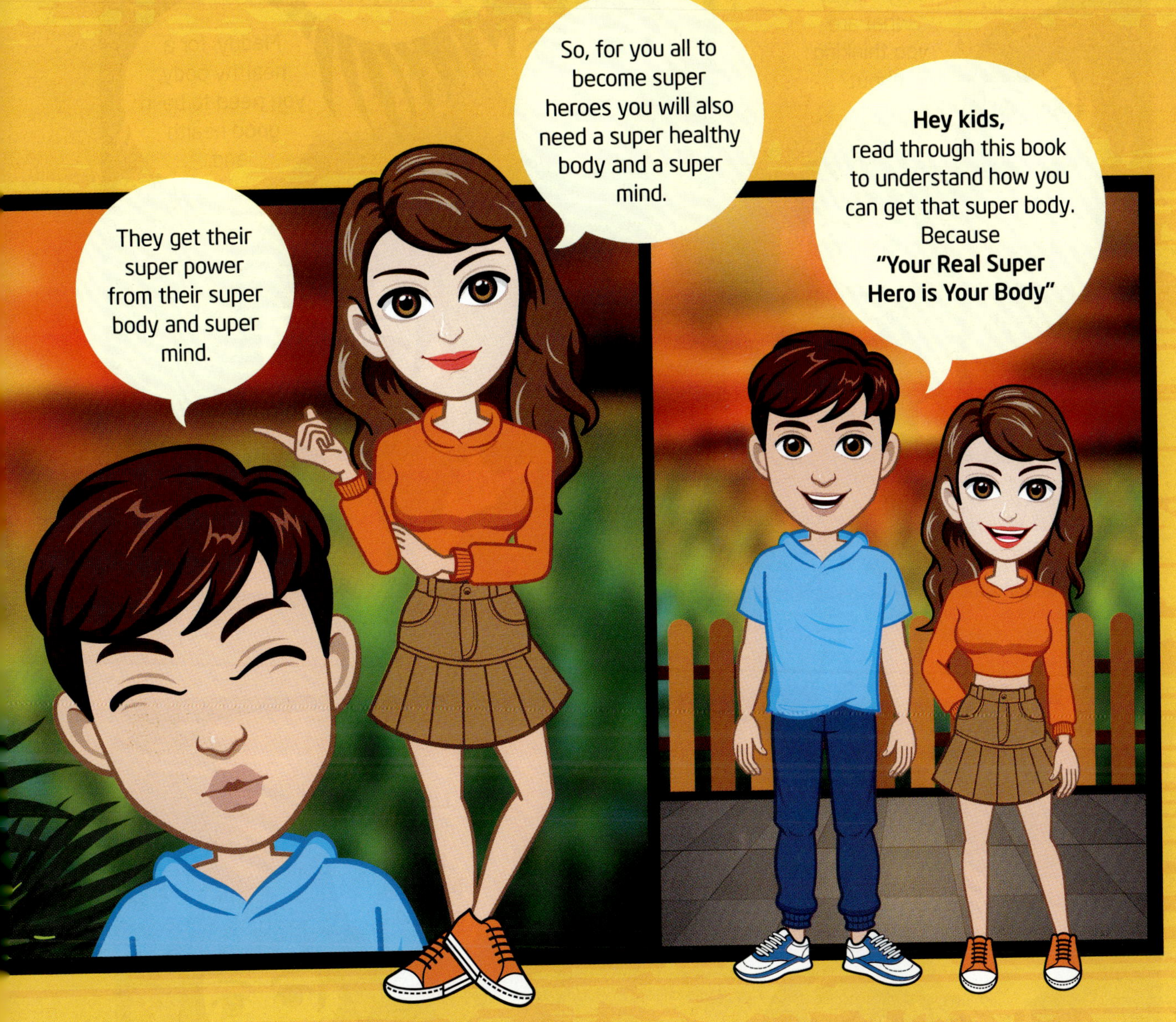

1. Introduction

Basic Nutrition

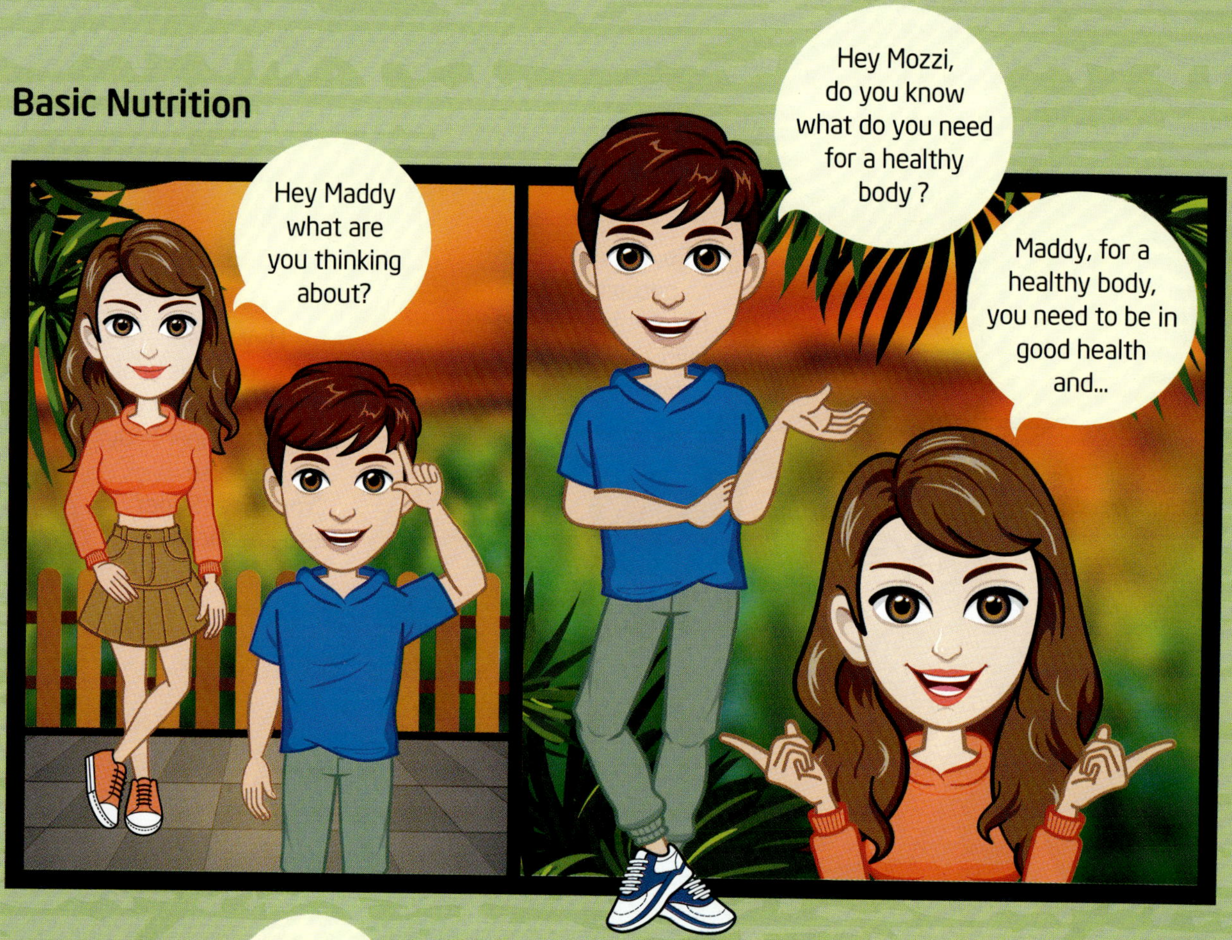

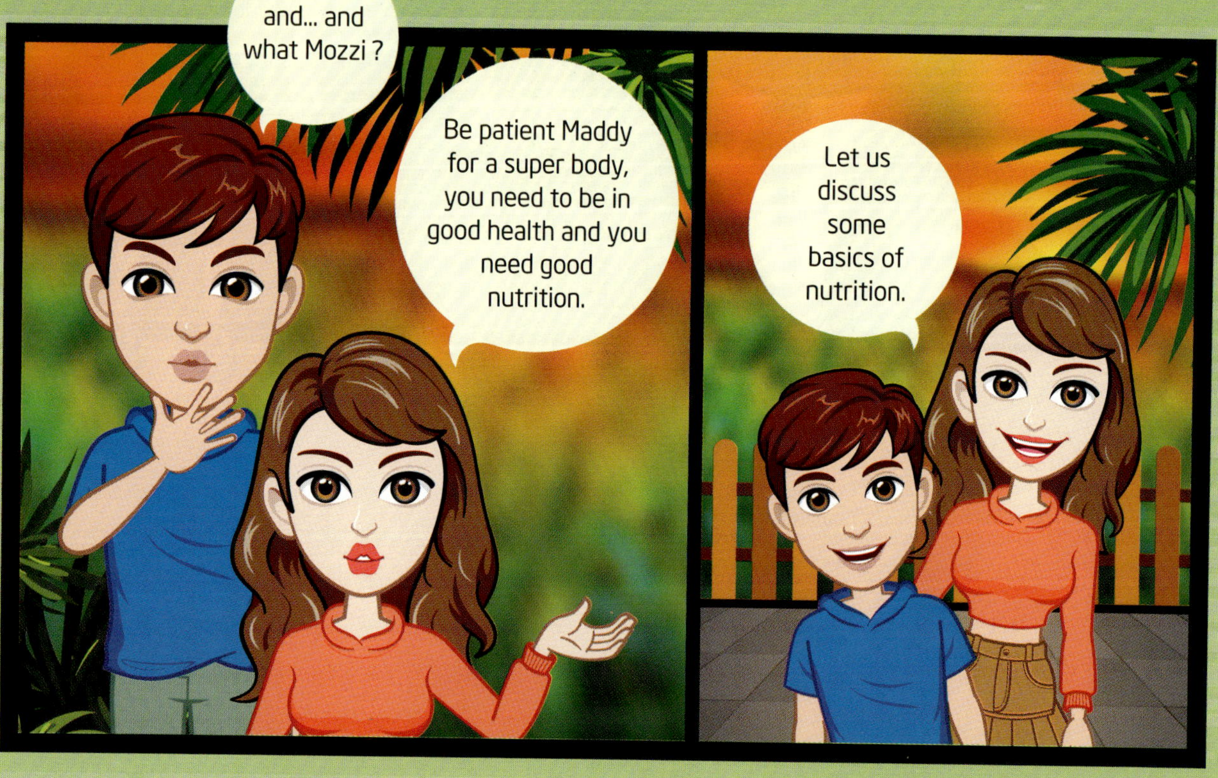

What is Health ?

Health is overall wellbeing. Health is dynamic balance of physical, mental and social wellbeing in adapting to different conditions of life and its environment.

What is Nutrition ?

Nutrition is defined as the scientific study of food and its relation to health. It is the science or study of proper balanced diet to promote health especially in human beings.

There are two nutritional statuses:

Good nutritional status: Good nutritional status means good immunity, shiny hair, glowing skin, sparkling eyes and a well-structured body. It is also reflected by his/her stamina and resistance to diseases.

Poor nutritional status : Poor nutritional status means poor physique, less stamina, dull hair, dull eyes, slumped posture, fatigue, and depression and poor sleep pattern. You may be overweight or underweight.

Have you ever seen any of these super heroes with a bad physique?

Just imagine Spiderman with a round tummy or Thor too weak to lift his hammer; they would never be able to do all the amazing things and save the world if they are not super fit!

What is a Food Pyramid ?

The Food Guide Pyramid is a recognizable nutrition tool that was introduced by the USDA in 1992. It is shaped like a pyramid to suggest that a person should eat more foods from the bottom of the pyramid and fewer foods and beverages from the top of the pyramid.

Food pyramid is based on following food groups

- Cereal and millets
- Body building foods
- Other vegetables and fruits
- Protective foods
- Energy foods.

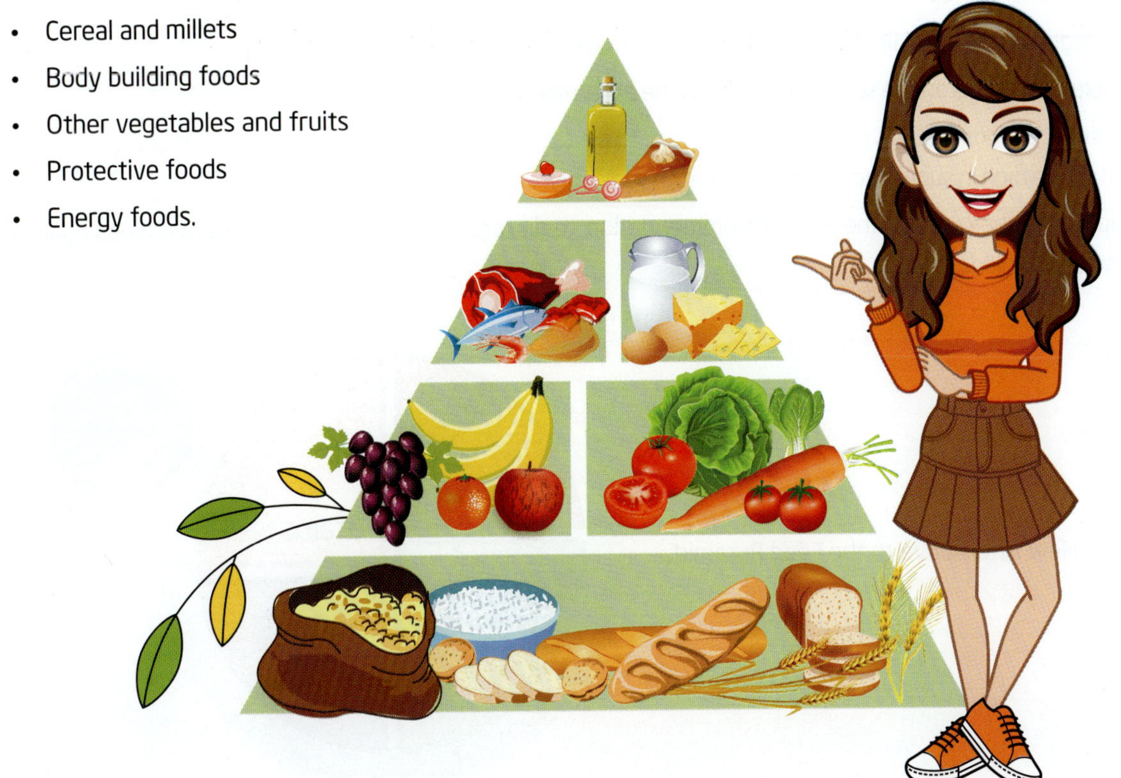

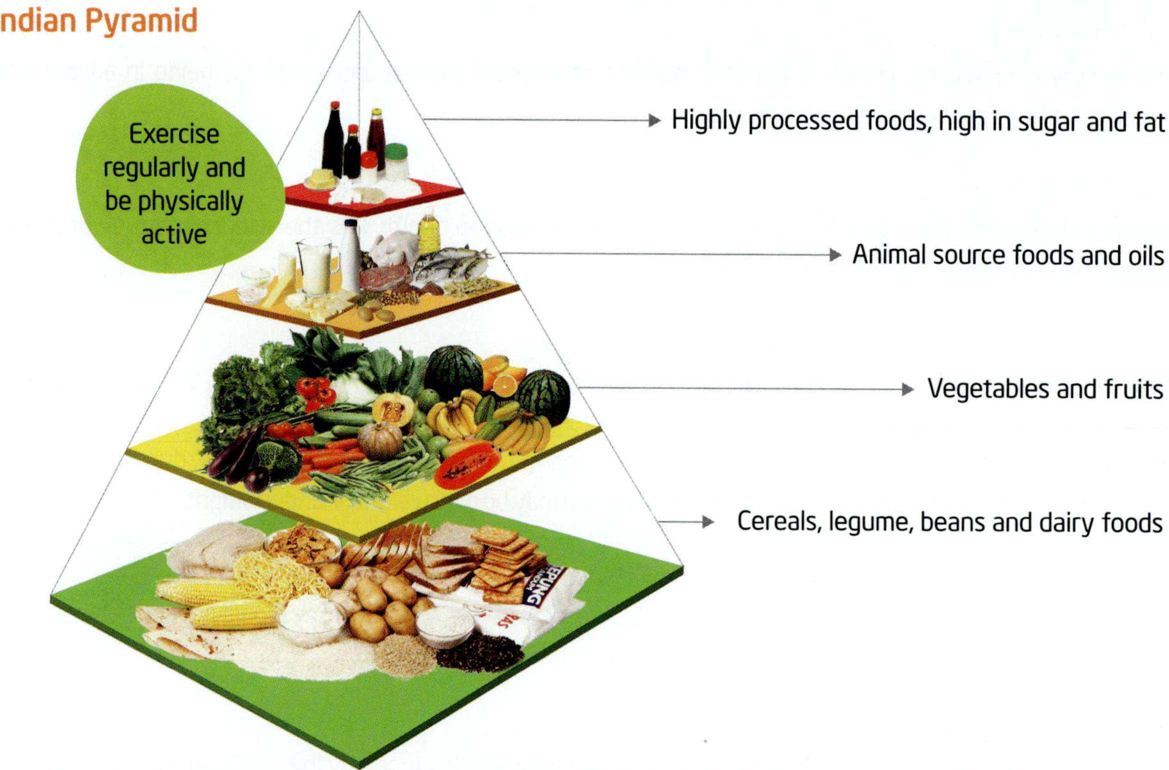

The dietary guidelines were launched in 1998. A revised version was published in 2011 and the updated guidelines was released in 2020. http:nin.res.in/RDA_Full_Report_2020.html.

The Indian adaptation of the Food Pyramid is divided into four levels of FOOD -

- Cereals, legumes/beans, dairy products at the base should be eaten in sufficient quantity;
- Vegetables and fruits on the second level should be eaten liberally;
- Animal source foods and oils on the third level are to be taken moderately; and at the apex, highly processed foods that are high in sugar and fat are to be eaten sparingly.
- Accompanying the pyramid there is a recommendation to do regular physical activity and warnings against smoking and drinking alcohol.

What is My Plate?
My Plate is a New Alternative to the Food Pyramid.

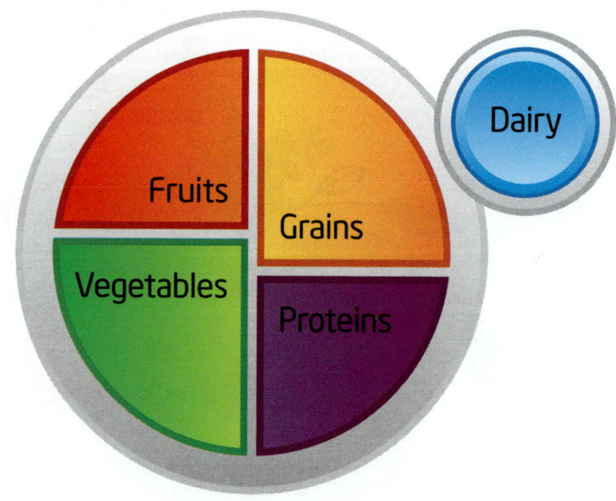

How Does My Plate Work?

The plate is divided into four sections to represent different food groups. Vegetables make up the largest section, followed by grains. Fruits and vegetables fill half the plate while proteins and grains fill the other half. A small blue circle on the side of the plate represents dairy.

How to plan Family Meals with My Plate?

My Plate is based on the 2015-2020 Dietary Guidelines for Americans, which provides detailed instructions for planning healthy meals and snacks.

- Make half your plate fruits and vegetables.

- Switch to 1% or skim milk, cheese, and other dairy options.

- Avoid full-fat dairy products.

- Half of your grains should be whole grains like jawar, bajra etc.

- Vary your proteins. Try different types, such as seafood, eggs, beans, unsalted nuts, lean meat and poultry.

- Watch out for sodium, saturated fat, and added sugars. For example, many fruit juices have little fruit and lots of sugar, and sweetened coffee drinks can contain a lot of sugar and fat. Try to drink water instead of sugary drinks.

- Be physically active Kids, especially, should have limited "screen time," and be encouraged to play outdoors rather than watching TV or using tablets.

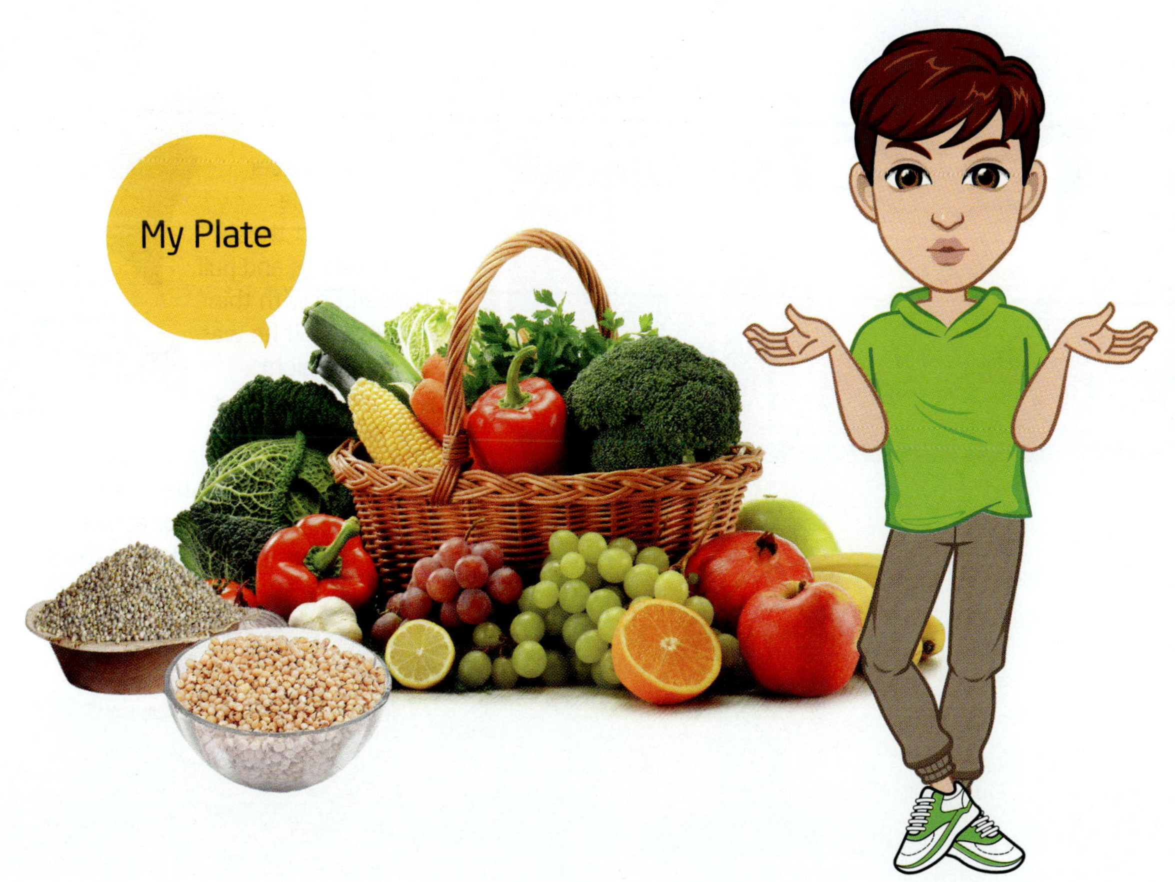

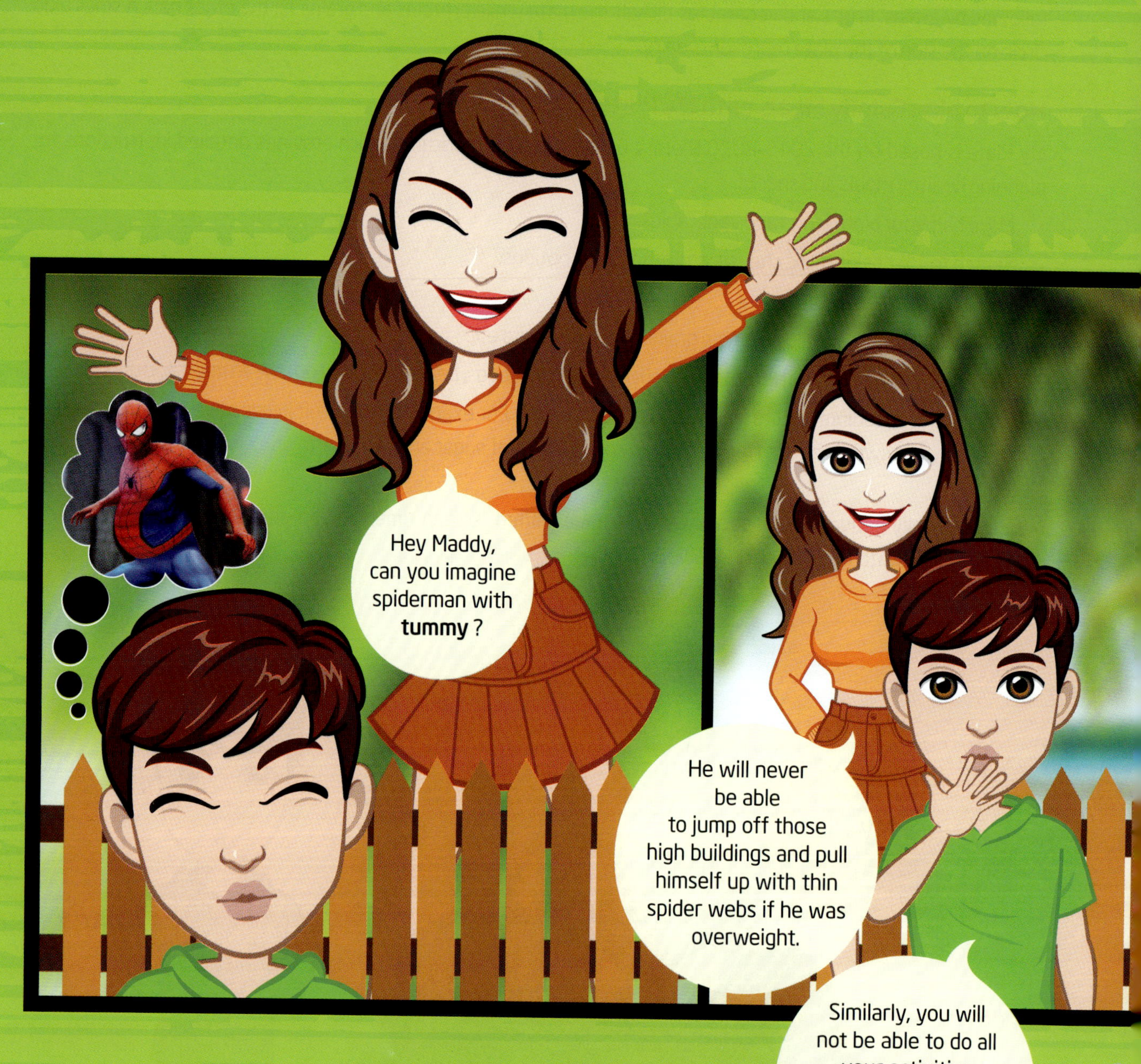
Hey Maddy, can you imagine spiderman with tummy ?
He will never be able to jump off those high buildings and pull himself up with thin spider webs if he was overweight.
Similarly, you will not be able to do all your activities throughout the day if you are not fit. You will feel dull and drained.

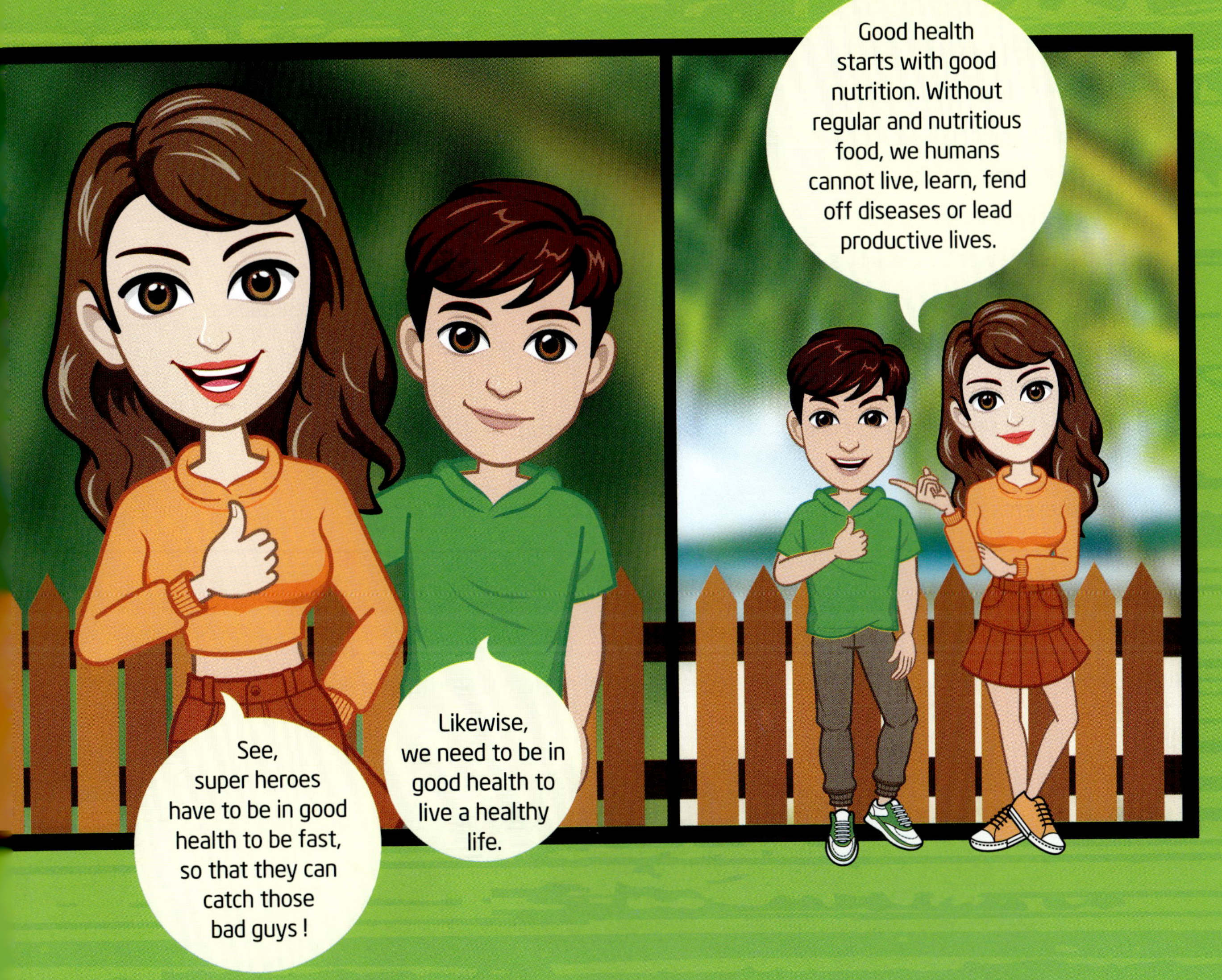

2. Good Health

What FAO (Food And Agricuiture Organisation Of The United Nation) Says ?

Good nutrition is our first line of defense against diseases and our source of energy to live and be active. Nutritional problems caused by an inadequate diet can be of many sorts, and when they affect a generation of youngsters, they can lower their learning capacities, thus compromising their future, perpetuating a generational cycle of poverty and malnutrition, with severe consequences on both individuals and nations. While young children are the most vulnerable to malnutrition, the right to adequate food is universal and good nutrition is essential for all. Problems of malnutrition – undernutrition, micronutrient deficiencies and obesity – exist in all countries and cut across socio-economic classes.

What are the GUIDELINES for GOOD HEALTH ?

- Maintain regularity in your routine.
- Eat as much natural food as you can.
- Consume seasonal foods as far as possible.
- Eat well, but do not overeat.
- Avoid excessive salt and spices.
- Avoid too many sweets, specially sugar.
- Eat food which contains carbohydrate, especially starch and fiber, for example fruits & vegetables.
- Avoid food that contain large amount of cholesterol and saturated fats like cheese & chips.
- Watch your weight and maintain ideal weight.
- Avoid eating the same kind of food all the time. Eat variety of foods.
- Drink a lot of water.
- Do regular exercise.

Suggestion Box

There is no term as a "Perfect Diet" for each individual. They are versatile and change according to the need and situation of each individual & there are variety of foods that supply different nutrition for good health.

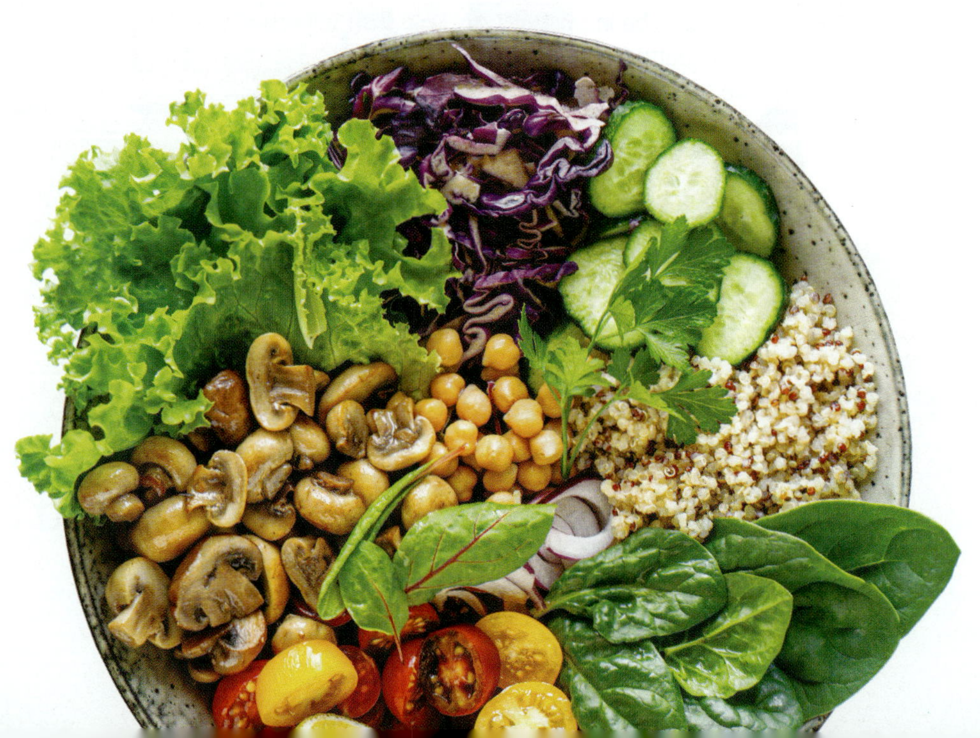

Good health is all about your, social, mental, and physical health. When you are happy and disease free then only one can say it's good health. Health depends on what kind of lifestyle you are following, and it includes your sleep pattern, your behavior with others, your social activity, your exercise pattern and a balanced diet. We can achieve good health through meditation, exercise and proper diet.

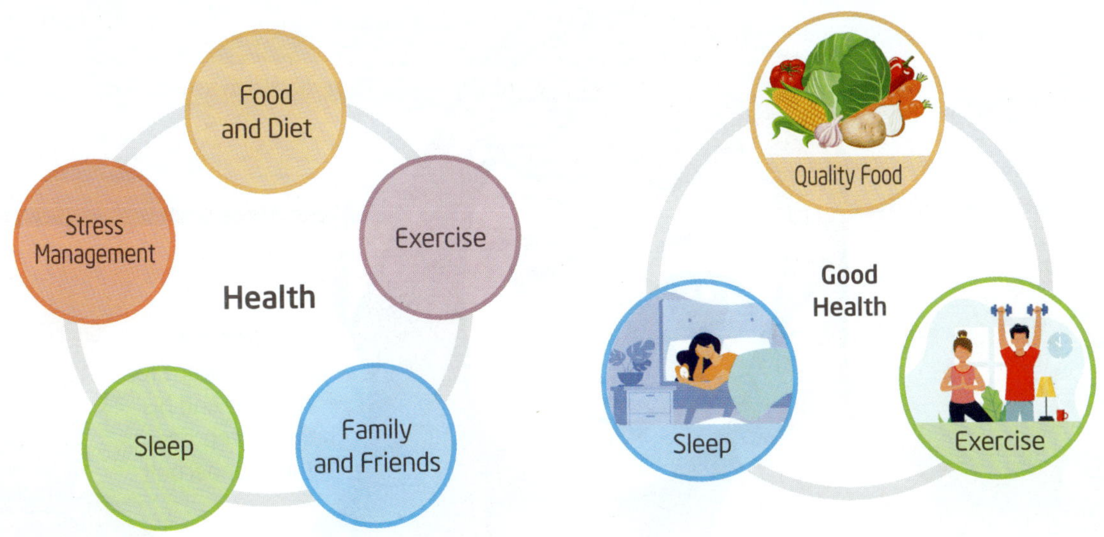

Suggestion Box

Energy

1. Be mindful while eating high fat and sugary food as it is high in calories and less in nutrients.
2. Keep moving every hour, it will help improve your metabolism and digestive system. For this, you can choose a short walk, jump, and other physical activities.
3. Try to do more walking, jumping, washing, cooking and other activities.
4. Use stairs instead of a lift.

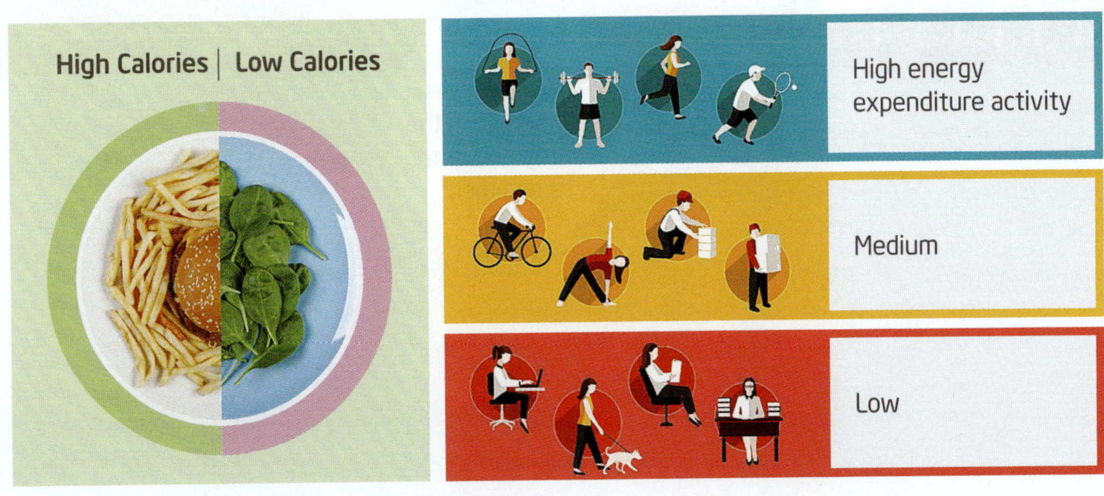

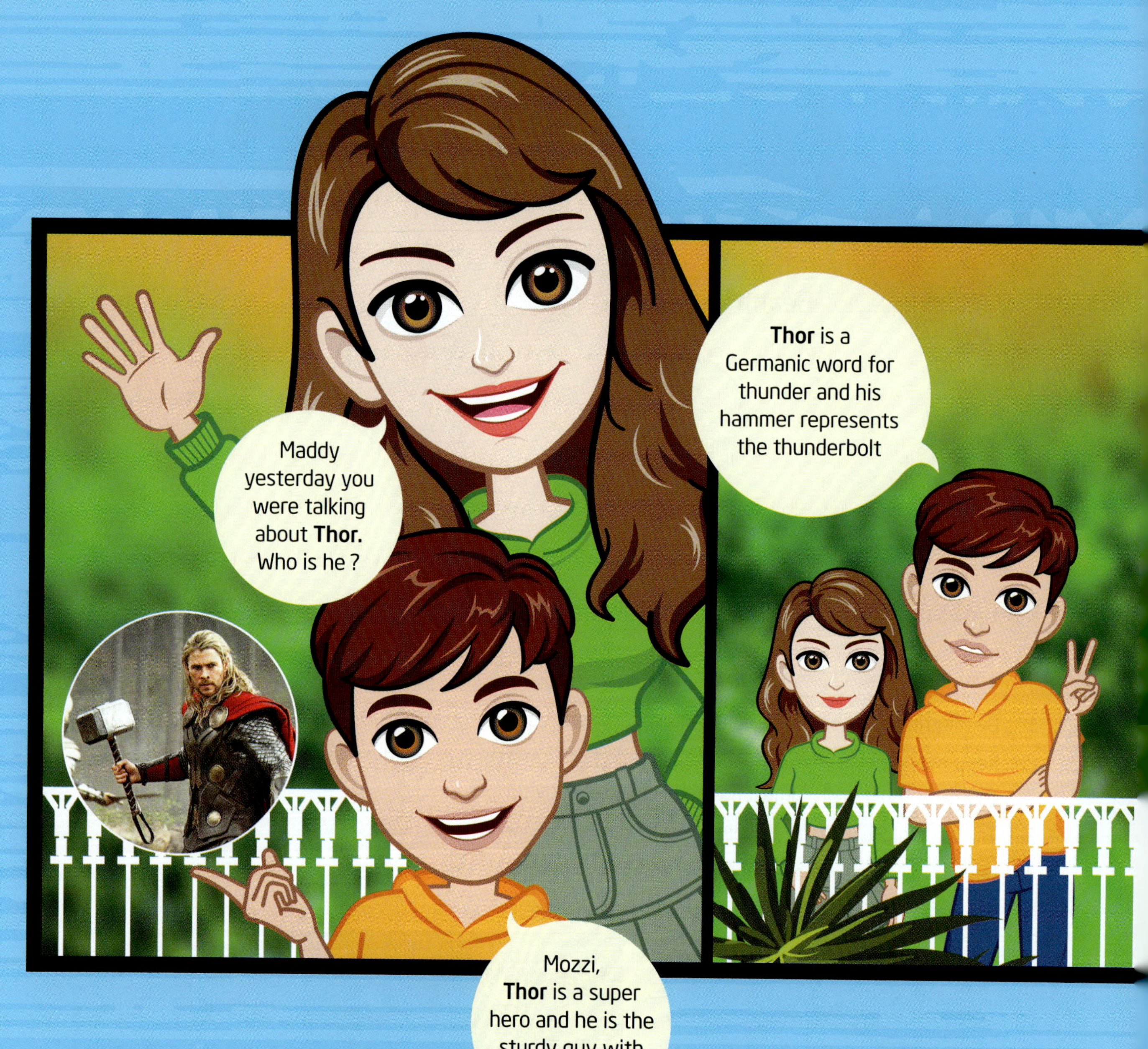

Maddy yesterday you were talking about **Thor.** Who is he ?
Mozzi, **Thor** is a super hero and he is the sturdy guy with a hammer.
Thor is a Germanic word for thunder and his hammer represents the thunderbolt

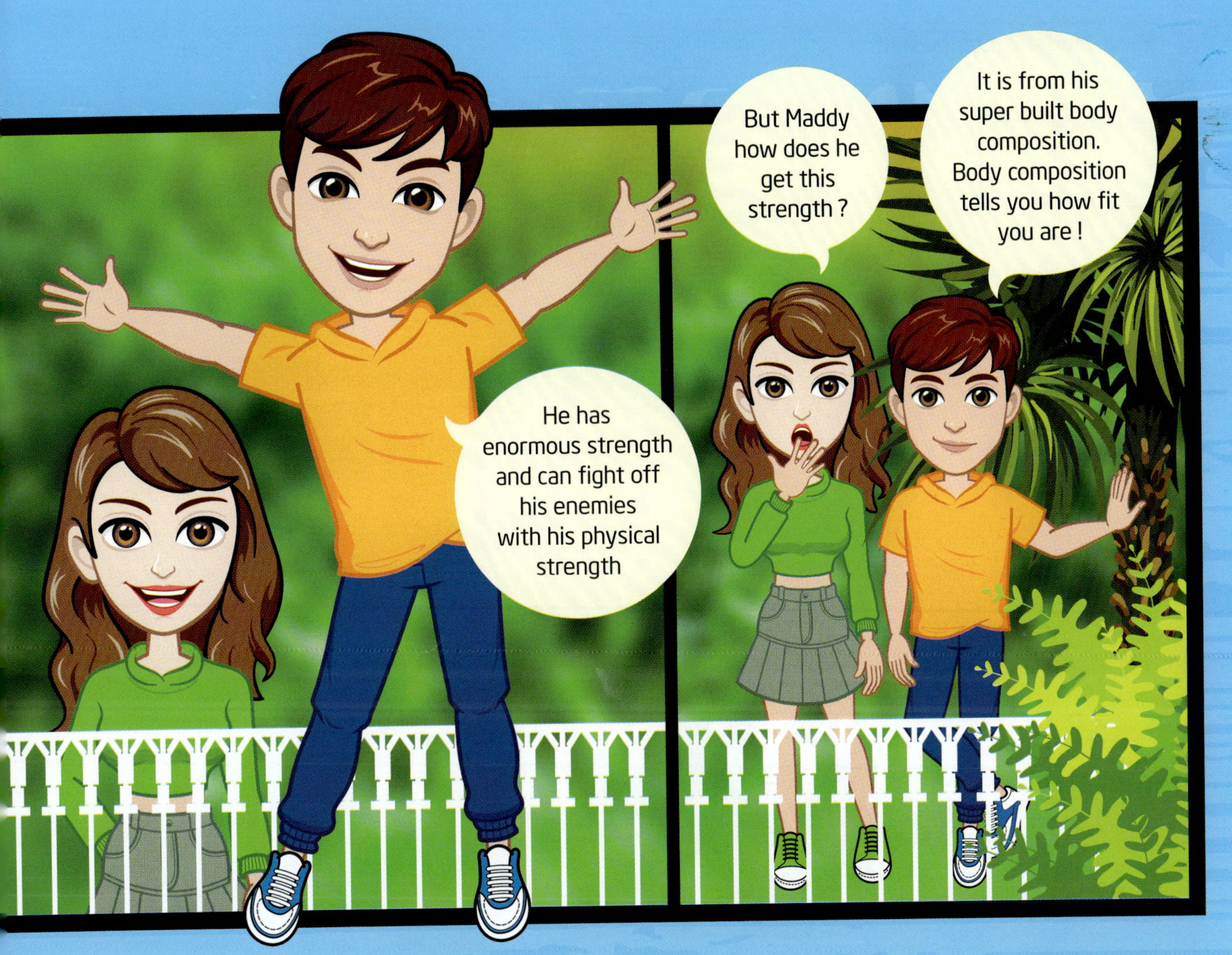

3. Body Composition

What is Body Composition?

The body is structurally made up of organs, bones, tissues and cells.

These in turn are made up of different chemical elements held together in varying combinations.

Several aspects of body composition, in particular the amount and distribution of body fat and the amount and composition of lean mass, are now understood to be important health outcomes in infants and children.

Following Table shows you our body is made up of lots of components:

Basic Model 2- Component		FAT		Fat-Free Mass (FFM)
N,K,Ca. Na	**Mineral**	**Fat**	**Other**
Carbon	Protein	ECS	Blood
Hydrogen	Fat	ECF	Bone
Oxygen	Water	Cell Mass	Adipose Tissue
			Skeletal
Atomic	Molecular	Cellular	Functional

Are you fit?

Check the growth chart to understand where you stand.

Average height and weight of boys at different ages

Age	Weight (kg)	Height (cm)
Birth	3.3	50.5
3 months	6.0	61.1
6 months	7.8	67.8
9 months	9.2	72.3
1 year	10.2	76.1
2 years	12.3	85.6
3 years	14.6	94.9
4 years	16.7	102.9
5 years	18.7	109.9
6 years	20.7	116.1
7 years	22.9	121.7
8 years	25.3	127.0
9 years	28.1	132.2
10 years	31.4	137.5
11 years	32.2	140.0
12 years	37.0	147.0
13 years	40.9	153.0
14 years	47.0	160.0
15 years	52.6	166.0
16 years	58.0	171.0
17 years	62.7	175.0
18 years	65.0	177.0

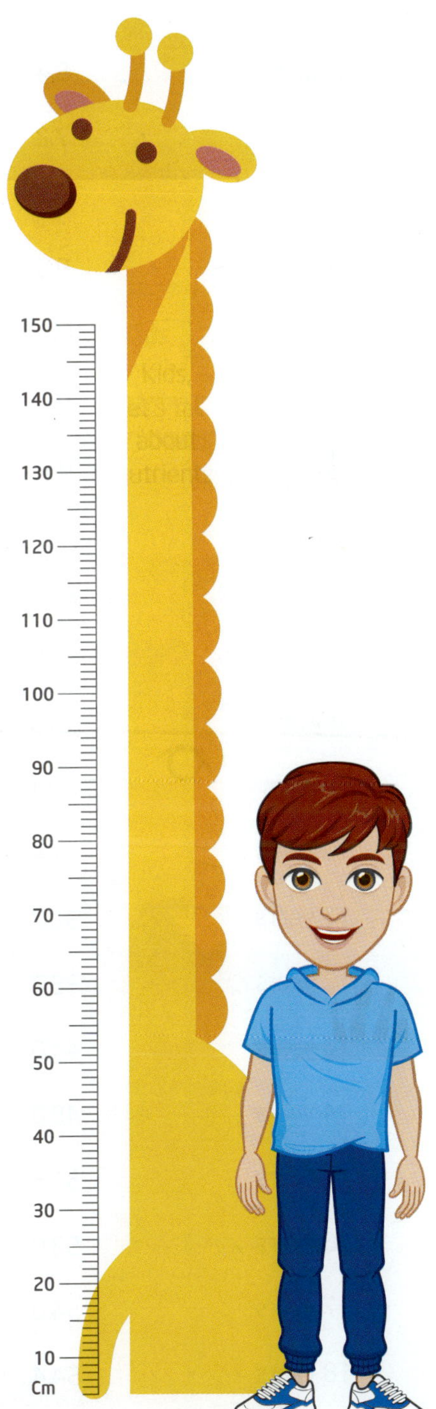

(Source: Nutrient Requirements and Recommended Dietary Allowances for Indians, I.C.M.R. 1990.)

Your Real Superpower Is Your Body

Are you fit?

Check the growth chart to understand where you stand.

Average height and weight of girls at different ages

Age	Weight (kg)	Height (cm)
Birth	3.2	49.9
3 months	5.4	60.2
6 months	7.2	66.6
9 months	8.6	71.1
1 year	9.5	75.0
2 years	11.8	84.5
3 years	14.1	93.9
4 years	16.7	102.9
5 years	18.7	109.9
6 years	20.7	116.1
7 years	21.8	120.6
8 years	25.3	127.0
9 years	28.1	132.2
10 years	31.4	137.5
11 years	32.2	140.0
12 years	38.7	148.0
13 years	44.0	150.0
14 years	48.0	155.0
15 years	51.5	161.0
16 years	53.0	162.0
17 years	54.0	163.0
18 years	54.4	164.0

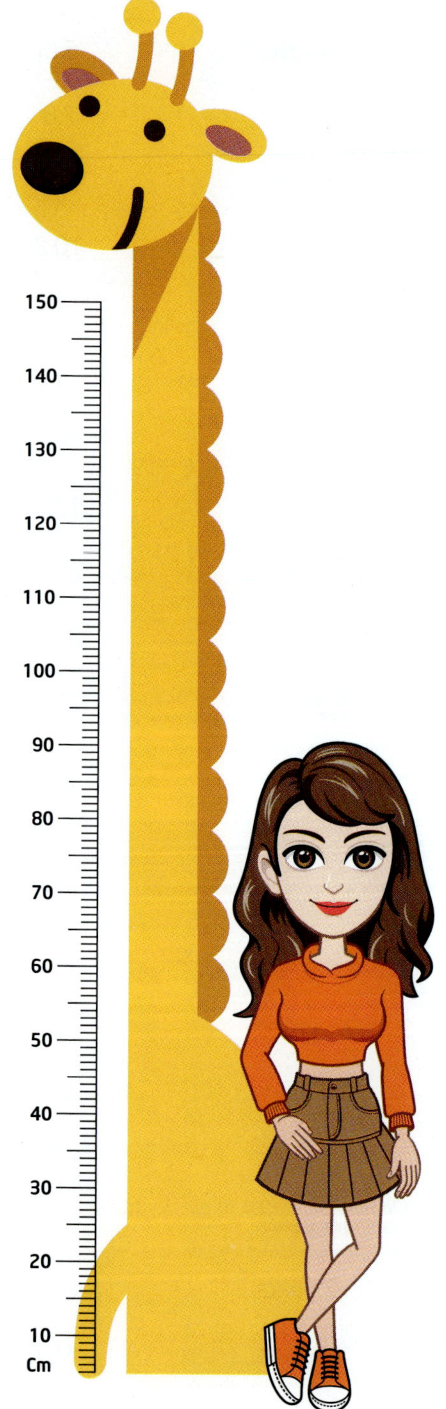

(Source: Nutrient Requirements and Recommended Dietary Allowances for Indians, I.C.M.R. 1990.)

What is Peak Height Velocity?

- It occurs at a mean age of 13.5 years in boys and 11.5 years in girls.
- Peak height velocity is 9.5 cm/y in boys and 8.3 cm/y in girls.
- Pubertal height gain averages 31 cm in boys and 29 cm in girls.

There are a number of variables that may directly or indirectly influence pubertal growth spurt including, gender, genetics, nutrition, endocrine regulation, physical activity and ethnicity. It is the interaction among several of these variables that may affect pubertal growth and maturation in complex ways.

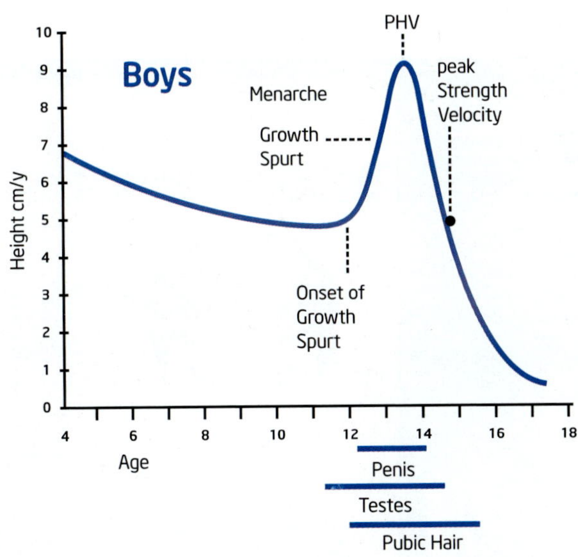

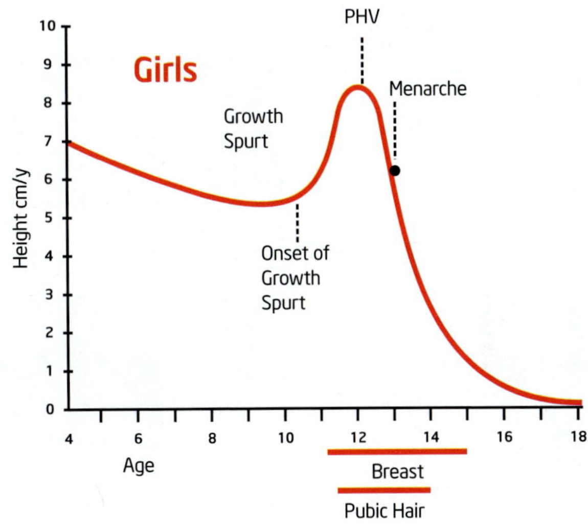

What You Can Do – To Improve Your PHV?

- Be active.
- Play sports or dance or do any physical activity for at least one hour daily.
- Eat a balanced diet.
- Add more protein to your diet.

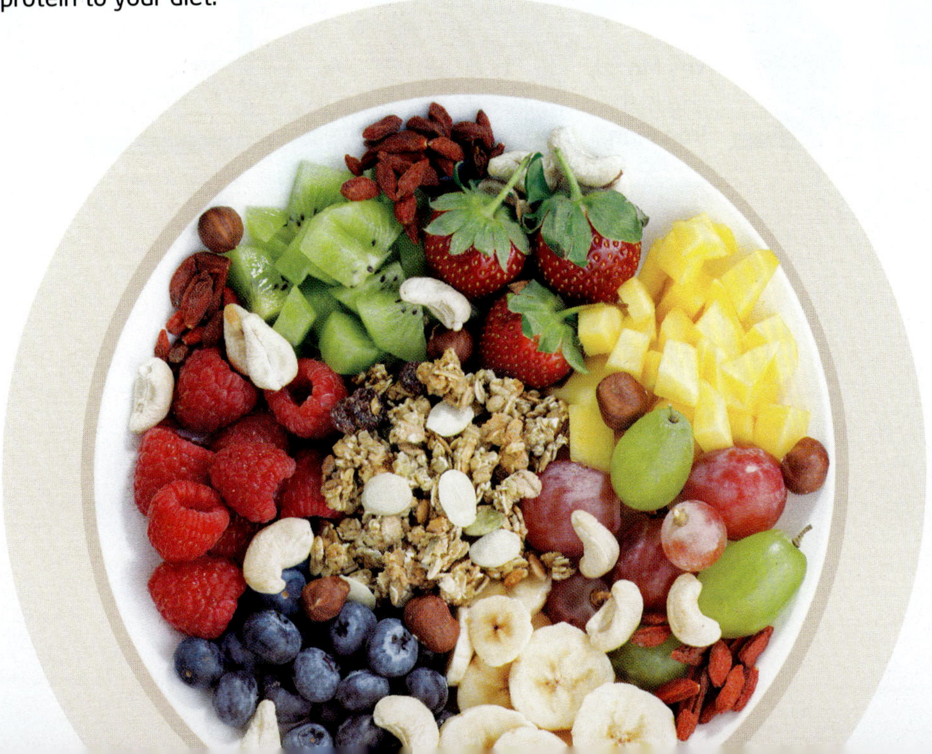

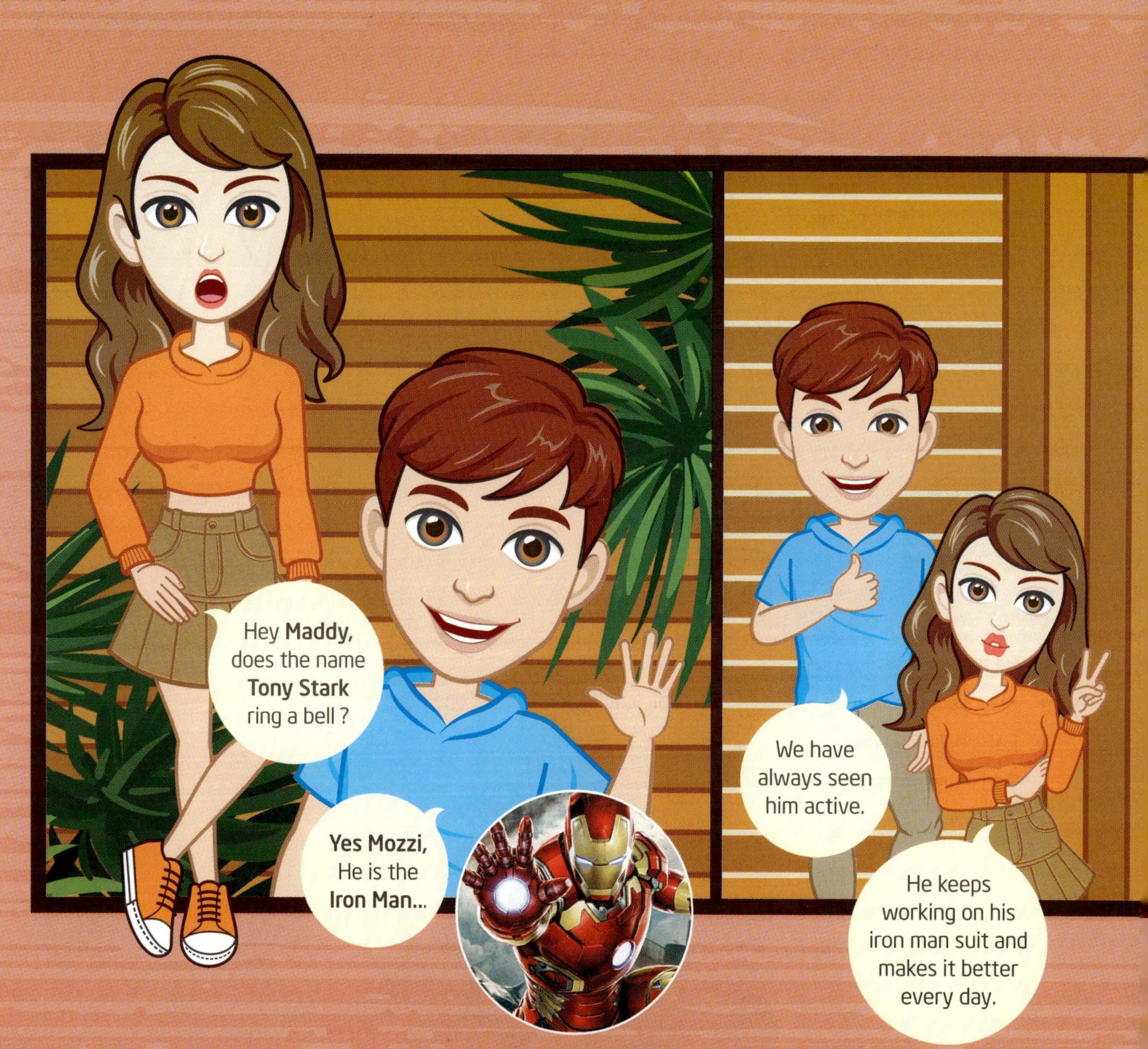

Hey Maddy, does the name Tony Stark ring a bell ?
Yes Mozzi, He is the Iron Man...
We have always seen him active.
He keeps working on his iron man suit and makes it better every day.

We will help you understand what Energy is and where does it come from.
I always wonder how does he manage to do it, even after fighting the bad guys so often ?
Well, the answer is simply Energy ! He is full of energy !

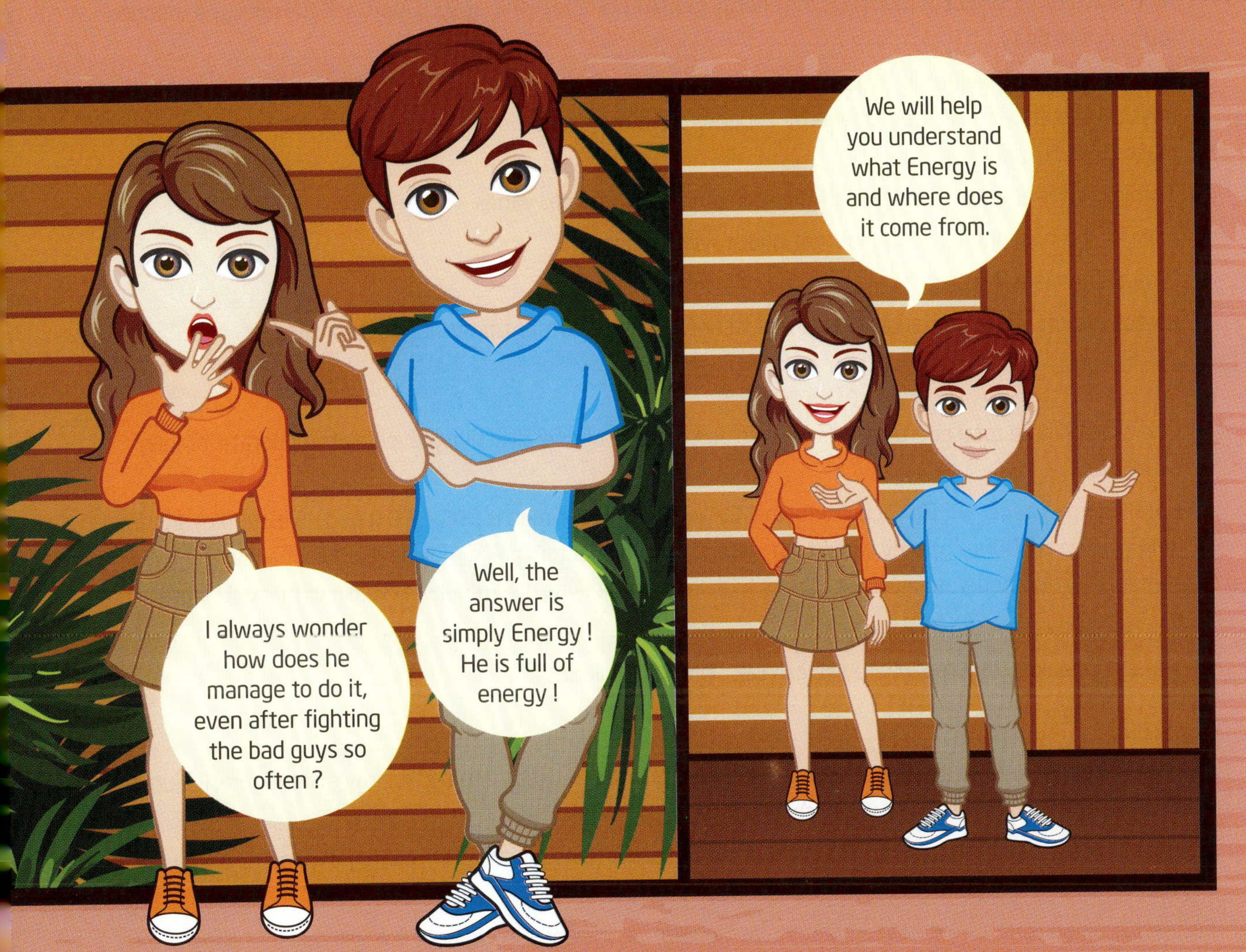

4. Energy

What is Energy ?

1. Energy is needed by the body to stay alive, grow, keep warm and move around.
2. Energy is provided by foods and drinks. It comes from fats, carbohydrates, proteins and fruit juices which the diet contains.
3. Energy requirements vary from one individual to the next, depending on factors such as age, gender, and body composition and physical activity level.
4. Energy expenditure is the sum of the basal metabolic rate (the amount of energy expended while at complete rest), the thermic effect of food (TEF, the energy required to digest and absorb food) and the energy expended in physical activity.
5. To maintain body weight, it is necessary to balance the energy derived from food with that expended in physical activity. To lose weight, energy expenditure must exceed intake, and to gain weight, energy intake must exceed expenditure.
6. The amount of energy that each of these macro nutrients provides varies

- Fats are the most energy dense nutrient, and provides 9kcal /g.
- Proteins provides 4 kcal /g.
- Carbohydrates (starch and sugars) are the least energy dense nutrient, providing just 4 kcal /g.

How to calculate your need of energy ?

- One can estimate total energy needs from an assessment of overall activity level (high, moderate, or low) as follows:

A) Basal energy needs = RMR x activity factor, B) where RMR for men is 900 + 10 x body weight (kg) and for C) RMR women is 800 + 7 x body weight (kg), and D) activity factors are E) low levels 1.2 of activity (sedentary), F) for moderate level 1.4, G) for high levels of activity 1.6 (regular exercise or manual labor).

- You can calculate by smart watch.
- You can download any app where you can calculate your calories.

Intake versus Expenditure

In order for people to maintain proper body weight, energy intake must be equal to energy expenditure. Failure to maintain energy balance results in weight change

Energy balance can be maintained by regulating energy intake (through the diet), energy expenditure (adjusting physical activity level to match intake) or a combination of both.

Failure to compensate an increase in energy intake with an increase in expenditure will result in weight gain (positive energy balance); conversely a reduction in energy intake which isn't matched by a reduction in physical activity levels will result in weight loss (negative energy balance).

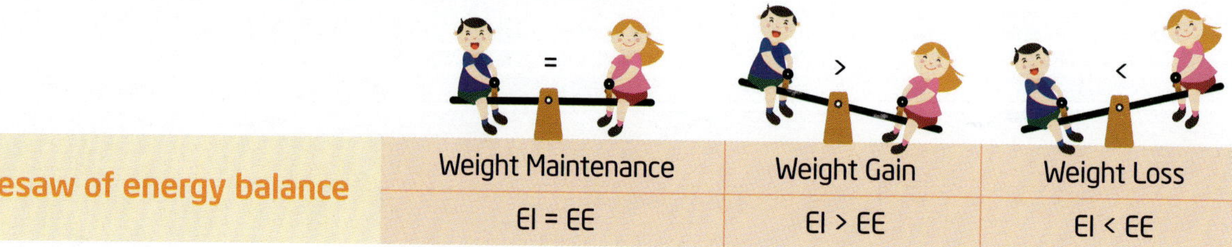

Seesaw of energy balance	Weight Maintenance	Weight Gain	Weight Loss
	EI = EE	EI > EE	EI < EE

● EE = Energy Expenditure, ● EI = Energy Intake

Energy requirement for children

Group	Particulars	Body Weight Kg	Net Energy g/day	Protein g/day	Visible fat g/day	Calcium mg/d	Iron mg/d
Mom	Sedentary Work	60	2320	60	25	600	17
	Moderate Work		2030		30		
	Heavy Work		3490		40		
Woman	Sedentary Work	55	1900	55	25		21
	Moderate Work		2230				
	Heavy Work		2850				
	Pregnant Woman		+350	+23	30	1200	35
	Lactation 0-6 month		+600	+19	30	1200	21
	6-12 month		+520	+13	30		
Infants	0-6 month	5.4	92Kcal/Kg/d	1.16g/Kg/d	-	500	46g/Kg/day
	6-12 month	8.4	50Kcal/Kg/d	1.169g/Kg/d	19		5
Children	1-3 year	12.9	1060	16.7	27	600	09
	4-6 year	18	1350	20.1	25		13
Children	1-3 year	12.9	1060	16.7	27	600	16
	4-6 year	18	1350	20.1	25		13
	7-9 year	12.9	1690	29.5	30		16
Boys	10-12 year	34.3	2190	39.9	35	800	21
Girls	10-12 year	35.0	2010	40.4	35	800	27
Boys	13-15 year	47.6	2750	54.3	45	800	32
Girls	13-15 year	46.6	2330	51.9	40	800	27
Boys	16-17 year	55.4	3020	61.5	50	800	28
Girls	16-17 Year	52.1	2440	55.5	35	800	26

Summary source - RDA for India 2010

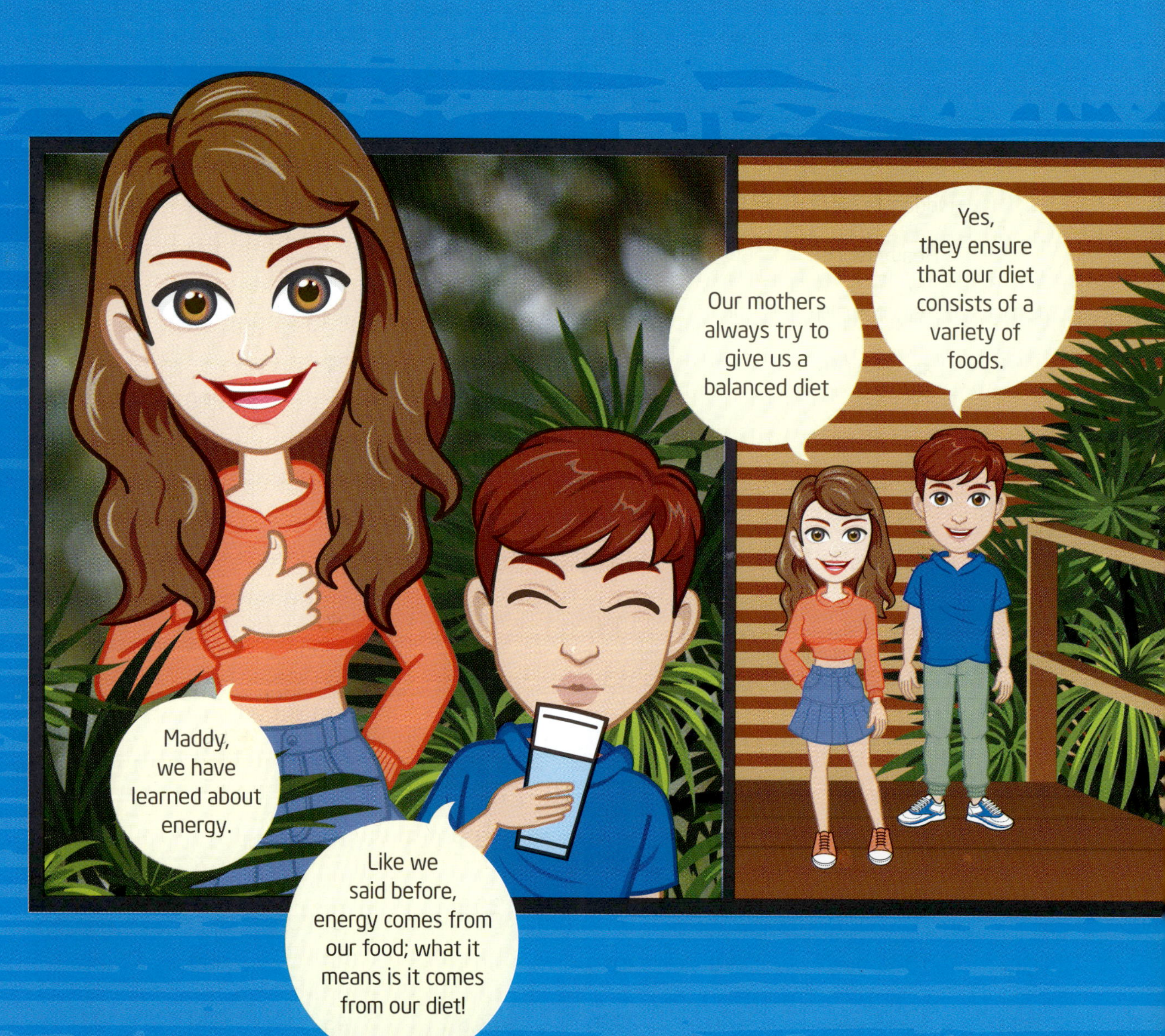

Maddy, we have learned about energy.
Like we said before, energy comes from our food; what it means is it comes from our diet!
Our mothers always try to give us a balanced diet
Yes, they ensure that our diet consists of a variety of foods.

That food provides us adequate amount of nutrients necessary for our good health.
But do you know what nutrients really are ?
Kids, let's talk about nutrients.

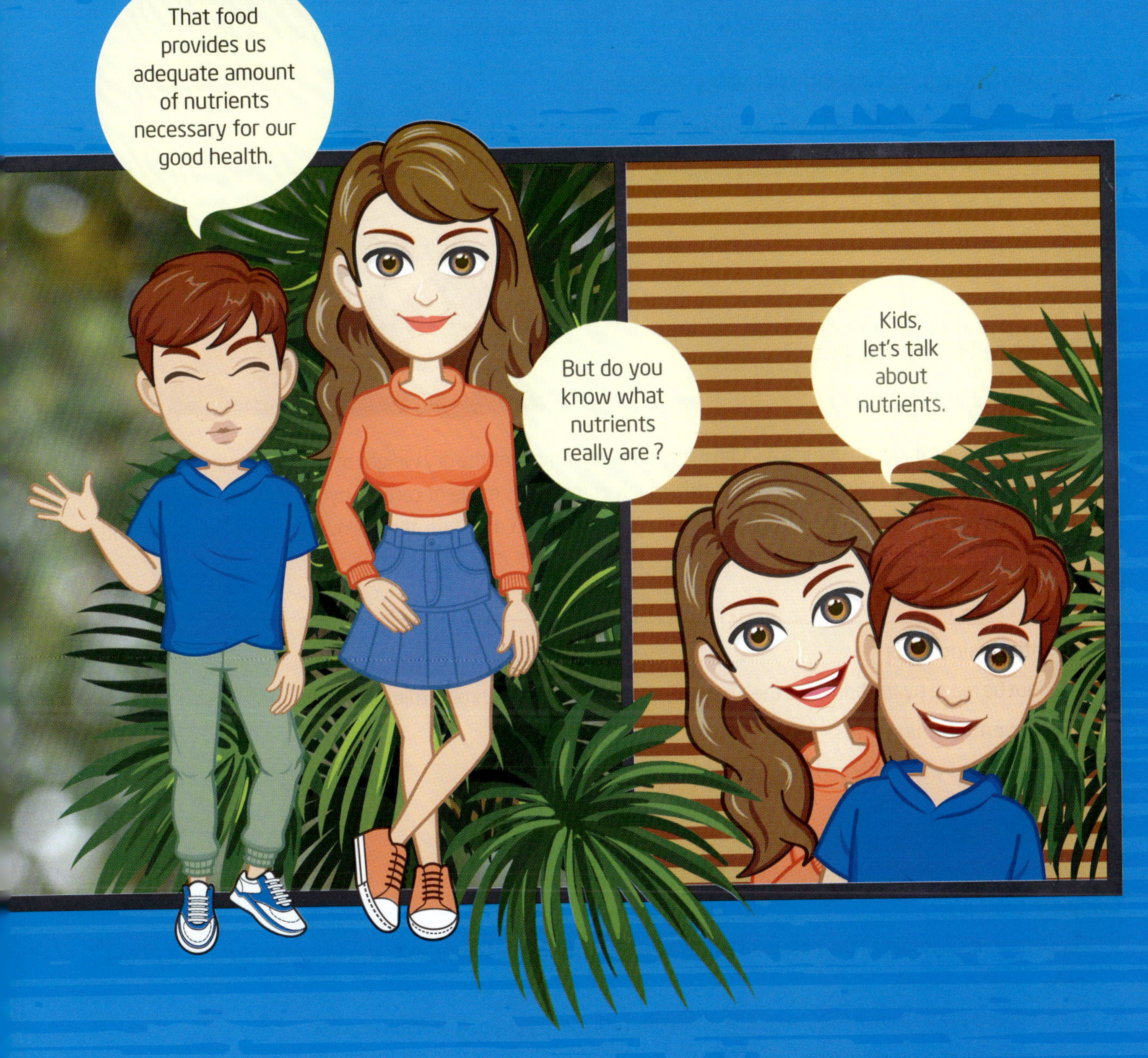

5. Nutrients

What are Nutrients ?

Nutrients are chemical components of food that supply nourishment to the body. They are required by the body in right amount and they must be eaten regularly. Each nutrient — Proteins, Carbohydrates, Fats, Minerals, Vitamins and Water perform a specific function in our body. They help us supply energy to the body, build and repair body tissues and regulate body processes.

Nutrients can be classified as follows

* Macronutrients - Proteins, Carbohydrates, Fats

* Micronutrients - Vitamins and Minerals

* Water and fiber

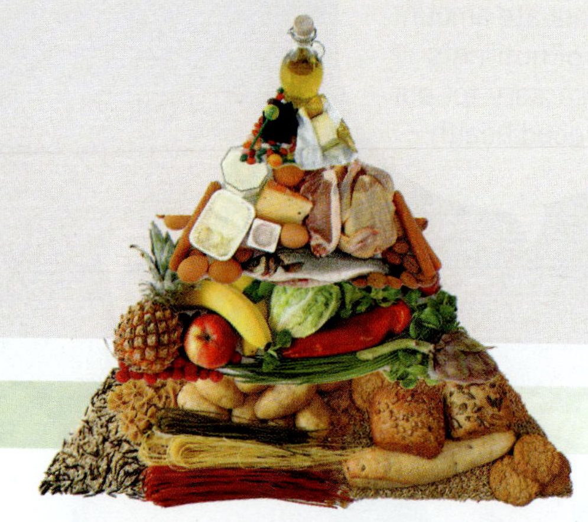

What are Macronutrients ?

1. Proteins

Proteins make up the major structure of all living cells and form most of the dry weight of the body cells. Chemically, proteins are composed of amino acids, which are organic compounds made of carbon, hydrogen, nitrogen, oxygen or sulfur. According to the National Institute of Health (NIH), amino acids are the building blocks of proteins and proteins are the building blocks of muscle mass.

There are two types of amino acids

* **Essential amino acids –**

They cannot be made by the body and their requirement has to be met through dietary intake.

* **Non - Essential amino acids –**

They can be made by the body and they need not be supplied through diet.

Sources of Proteins

We should consider the type of proteins while thinking about the sources of proteins.

Complete proteins –

* These proteins contain all the essential amino acids in sufficient quantity and ratio to supply the needs of the body.

* Such proteins are of animal origin e.g.- milk and milk products, eggs, poultry, meat and fish.

* The quality of proteins is superior.

Incomplete proteins –

* These proteins contain one or more of the essential amino acids and therefore they do not support life on their own.

* All plant sources are an example of this protein and that's why we need to combine it.

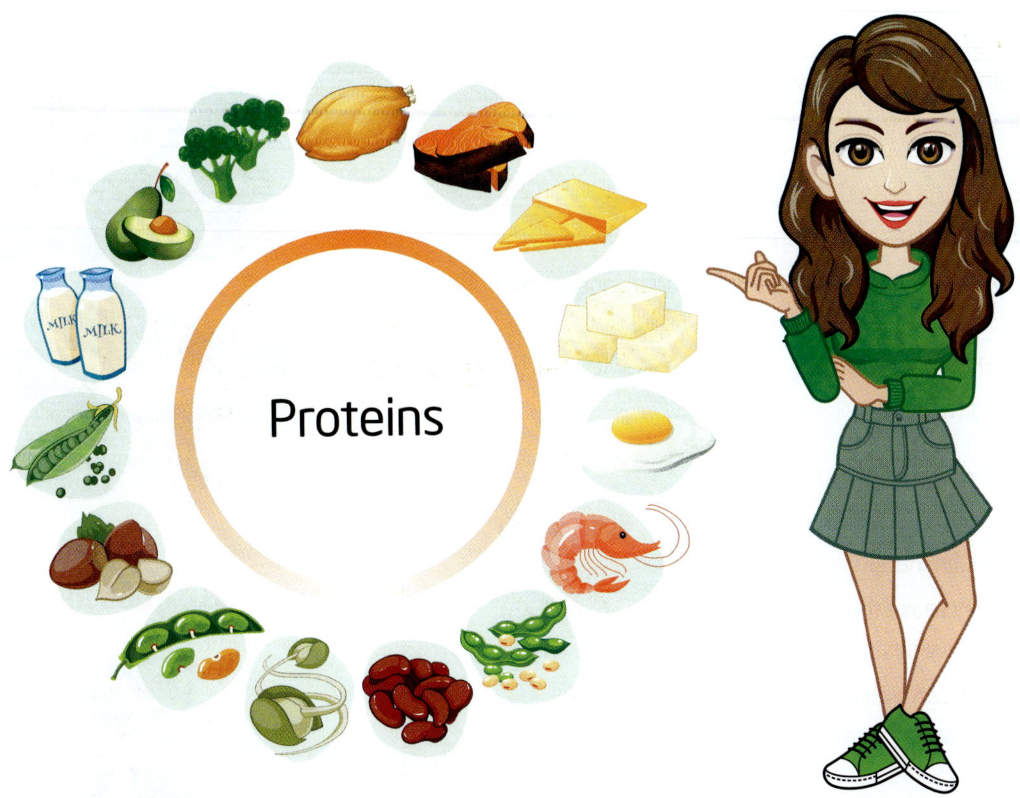

Functions of Proteins

- Proteins are present in all the living cells of our body and are required for growth and maintenance.
- It is required for highly specialized function in our body such as :
- Supply of energy.
- It helps the immune system stay strong.
- It also helps you to stay full.
- Deficiency of protein can cause weight loss, anemia, reduced resistance to infections, impaired wound healing, loss of hair, change in texture of hair and fatigue.

How to calculate the Proteins?

Total protein = 1 gm X ideal weight.
Recommended value of daily requirement of protein is 1 gm per body weight.

Suggestion Box

- Eat rajma/ chola or sprouts instead of dal.
- Always make combination of cereal and pulses like idli, khichadi, dal chawal, chola paratha the reason being some amino acids are present in cereals and some amino acids are present in pulses. So a combination gives you complete amino acids.
- Eating high biological proteins every day is very important as it has all essential as well as non-essential amino acids e.g all animal food (egg, fish, chicken), milk and milk products (cheese, curd, paneer), soybean.
- Nuts and seeds also have good amount of proteins, so don't miss it.

2. Carbohydrates

It is the main source of energy and almost 70% of our food carbohydrates.

Sources of Carbohydrates

There are two kind of carbohydrates

Simple carbohydrates –They come from sugar, jaggery and honey.

Complex carbohydrates –They come from grains, cereals, fruits and vegetables.

Functions of Carbohydrate

- Complex carbohydrates make fecal bulk which facilitates elimination.
- They also increase the good bacteria which are present in our digestive system.
- They alone can work as a source of energy for the central nervous system.

Excess of carbohydrates can cause

- Increase in the incidence of dental caries.
- Obesity.
- Irritation of the gastro intestinal tract.
- Depressed appetite (If empty calories such as those found in synthetic soft drinks are consumed).

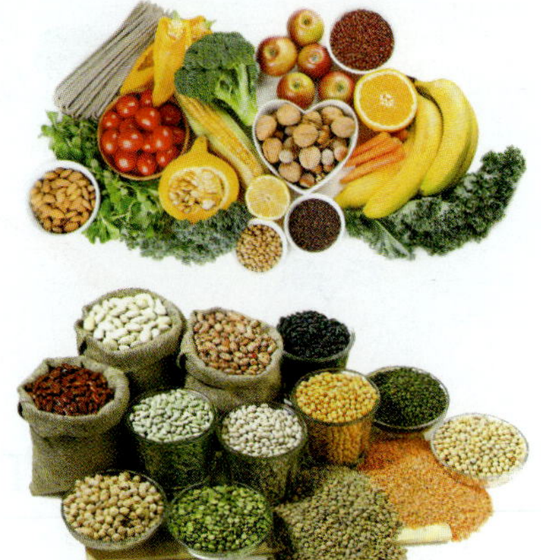

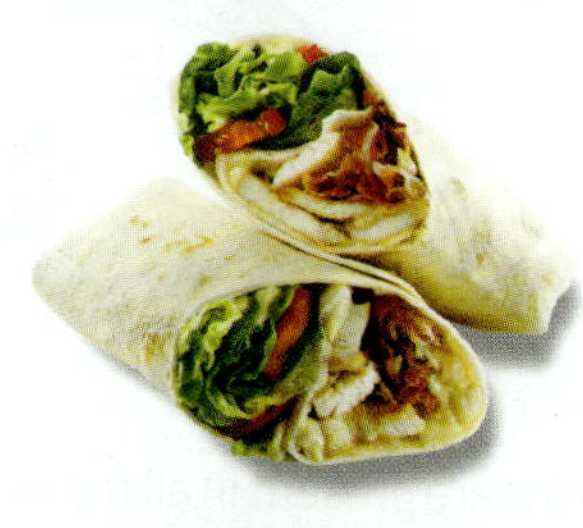

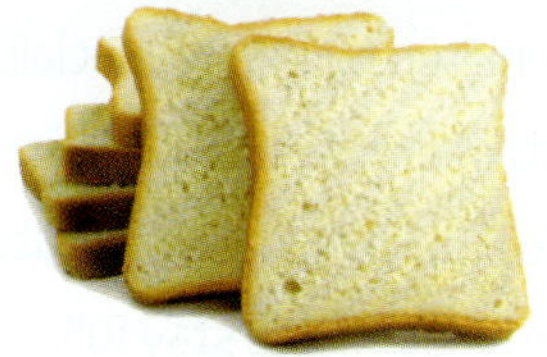

Suggestion Box

- Eat less refined flour.
- Say no to highly sugary food products.
- Do not add sugar to your drinks.
- Do not add sugar in your milk because milk is a good source of calcium and sugar interfers with the absorption of calcium.
- Prefer raw honey or chemical free jaggery.
- Avoid soft drinks and tetra pack fruit juices.
- Avoid bakery food products and biscuits which are made up of maida or refined sugar.
- Avoid pizza, burger and pasta which are made up of refined flour.
- Avoid cakes, pastries and other sweets.

3. Fats

Fats are more concentrated form of storage of energy than carbohydrates. In the presence of an adequate supply of carbohydrate, fats get stored in the fatty tissues.

An excess of daily intake of carbohydrates also results in its conversion and storage, as fat in the fatty tissues. Hence an overweight person not only needs to avoid intake of fats but also avoid excessive amount of carbohydrates.

Fats are found in all foods. They improve consistency and tend to make food tastier.

1gm of fat produces 9 kcal, a higher value than those produced by carbohydrates and proteins. In a balanced diet they should represent 25% to 30 % of the daily food intake, with a constant presence of essential fatty acids.

Sources of Fats

They can be classified as –

- Visible Fats –Sources of these are oil, butter, meat and fish.
- Invisible Fats –Sources of these are meat, fish, cheese, eggs, olives and seeds.

Fatty acids in food can also be classified as –

Saturated Fatty Acids

- They don't have unsaturated carbon bonds.
- E.g. : Vanaspati ghee, milk cream, ice-cream, butter, cheese, egg yolk, chocolates, and rich desserts.
- We should limit saturated fats. Foods which have saturated fats are dangerous for our body.

Unsaturated Fatty Acids

- They have double carbon bonds and they are considered to be good fats.
- Monounsaturated – one double bond e.g. avocado, olives, olive oil, peanut butter, peanut oils, chicken, eggs, cashew fruits.
- Polyunsaturated - more than one double bond e.g. - Til (sesame seeds), fish, oil (soyabean, sunflower, groundnut oil).

Another way to classify fatty acids is

Essential fatty acids –

- They cannot be synthesized by the body.
- So, they are supplied through the diet.
- Many health disorders and especially those related to skin can be successfully managed through proper supply of the essential fatty acids.

Non-essential fatty acids:

- They can be synthesized by the body and need not be supplied through diet.

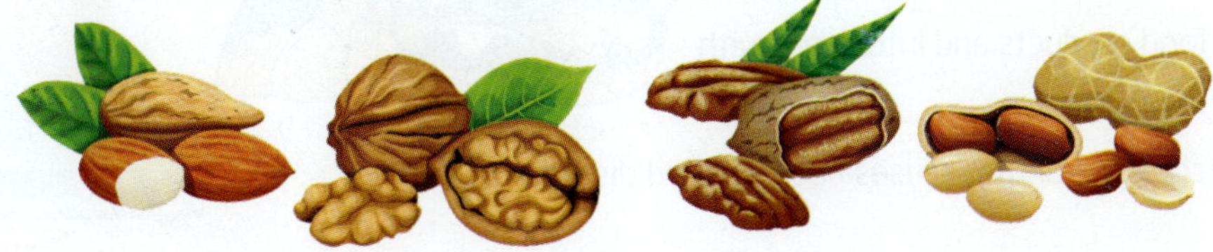

Cholesterol

Cholesterol is a fat like material found in cells of your body. Your body requires cholesterol to make hormones, vitamin D, and helps you to digest foods. Your body produces all the cholesterol it needs. Cholesterol is also found in foods from animal sources, such as egg yolks, meat, and cheese. The body needs cholesterol as It's a building block for human tissues, but when the cholesterol levels get too high, the fatty substance can accumulate in the blood vessels, which can cause serious health issues such as heart attacks, strokes, artery disease.

Hence maintaining the cholesterol level is important. Eating large amounts of saturated fat, trans fat and sugars can raise cholesterol levels. HDL (high-density lipoprotein, or good cholesterol) and LDL (low-density lipoprotein, or bad cholesterol) are two types of lipoproteins that are responsible for carrying cholesterol to and from the body's cells in the blood. HDL carries the bad cholesterol back to your liver, where it's broken down and eliminated from your body. LDL contributes to fatty buildups in arteries thus contributing to heart attacks.

The most common cause of high cholesterol is an unhealthy lifestyle such as unhealthy eating habits, lack of physical activities and smoking. You can maintain your cholesterol level by maintaining healthy lifestyle which includes healthy eating habits, regular exercise and weight management.

Trans Fatty Acids

Trans fat, also called trans-unsaturated fatty acids, is a type of unsaturated fats. Your body does not need any trans fats. Trans fat provides no health benefits. Instead, it is associated with a risk of developing many diseases. Eating these fats increase your risk for health problems such as high LDL, lower HDL, weight gain. Many high fat foods such as preservative foods and fried foods have a lot of trans fat.

Fat Fact

According to FSSAI, most of the processed food products and fast foods are rich in fat content which leads to onset of NCD-non communicable diseases like early age diabetes and obesity etc.

Functions of Fats

- Fats give high calories.
- Fats carry fat soluble vitamins A, D, E and K.
- Essential fatty acids are needed for the maintenance of body functions.
- Cholesterol is needed for synthesis of sex hormones.

Excess Fats in the Diet

- Can cause obesity.
- Abnormally slows down the digestion and absorption of food products and Interferes with the absorption of calcium.
- Increases bad cholesterol that causes heart related diseases.

- Eat limited amount of oil, butter, vanspati, cheese.
- Indian sweets as well as cakes have more fats, so avoid them.
- Eat fish, walnuts, seeds and nuts because they have good fats.
- Coconut oil should be used wisely.

DHA - Omega 3 fatty acids

Benefits of Omega 3 fatty acids:

- It is an essential fatty acid so needs to be taken through diet.
- It reduces LDL cholesterol which in turn reduces risk of heart attack.
- It also provides anti-inflammatory benefits.
- It is good for rheumatic arthritis.
- It reduces joint tenderness.
- It is good for Parkinson's disease and Alzheimer's disease.
- Extremely good for skin.

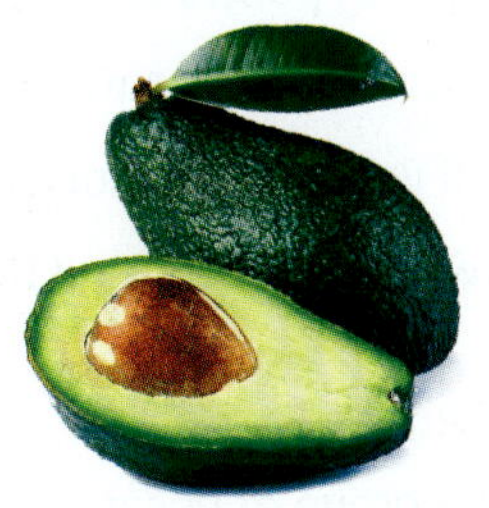

Fat Fact

DHA omega 3 fatty acid is beneficial for brain development of a child.

Sources of Omega 3 Fatty Acids:

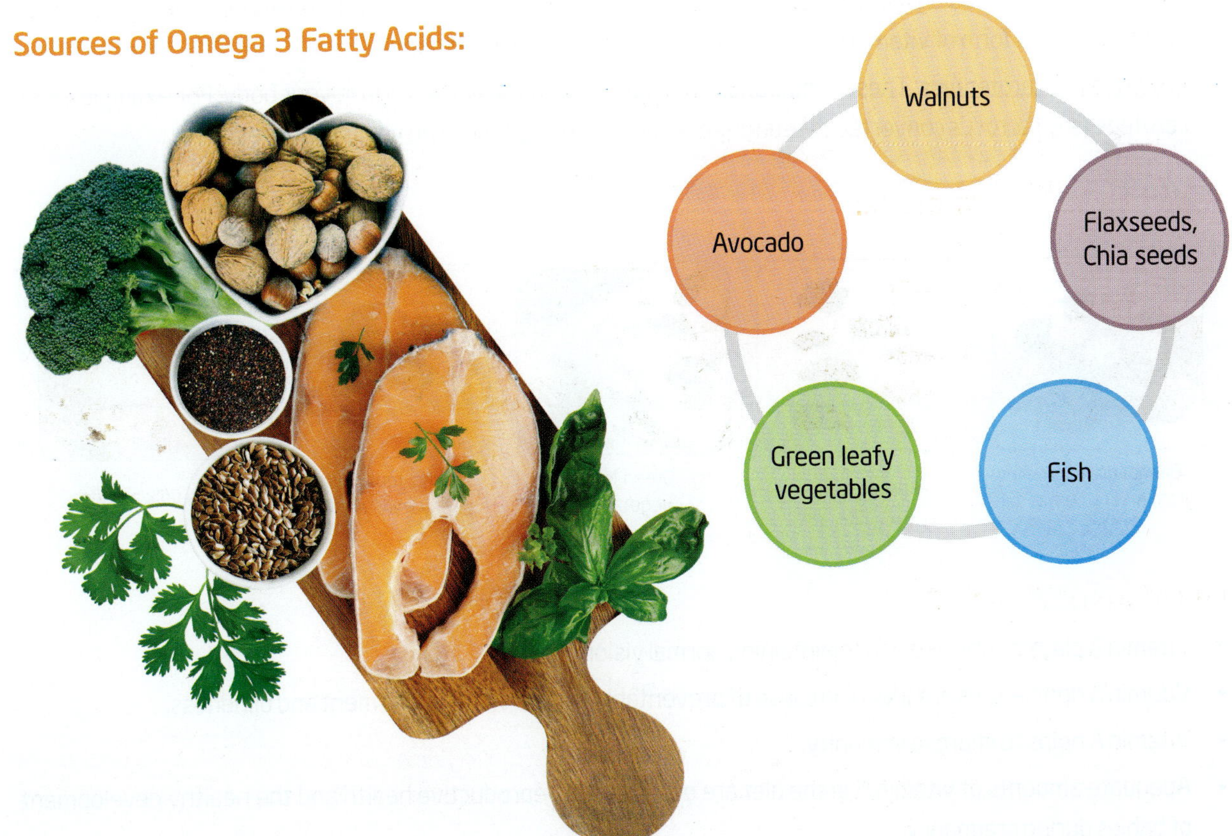

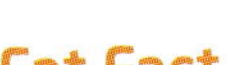

What are Micronutrients ?

Vitamins & Minerals are considered to be micronutrients. These are considered to be the powerhouse of our body. Vitamin and minerals make us stronger and hence are the real heroes of our body.

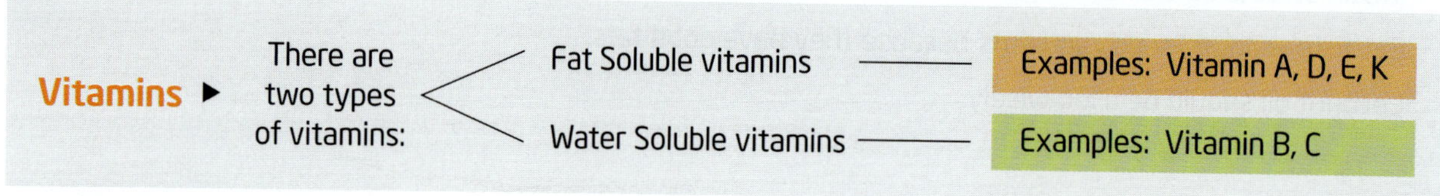

Couple of points to note:

- Avoiding fat from diet or taking less fat in diet can deprive you from fat soluble vitamins.
- If you perspire a lot while playing, then you need more water-soluble vitamins in addition to more water.

Now, let's understand these vitamins a little more.

Vitamin A

It is a group of unsaturated nutritional organic compounds that includes retinol, retinal, retinoic acid, and several provitamin A carotenoids (Most notably beta-carotene).

Sources of Vitamin A

Vitamin A can be found in two principal forms in foods.

- Preformed Vitamin A: It is known as the active form of the vitamin, which your body can use as it is. It is found in animal products including meat, chicken, fish and dairy and includes the compounds retinol, retinal and retinoic acid. Retrino the form of vitamin A absorbed when eating animal food sources.
- Provitamin A carotenoids: These compounds are converted to the active form in your body. For example, beta-carotene (e.g. carrot) is converted to retinol (an active form of vitamin A) in your small intestine.

Food rich in Beta carotene:

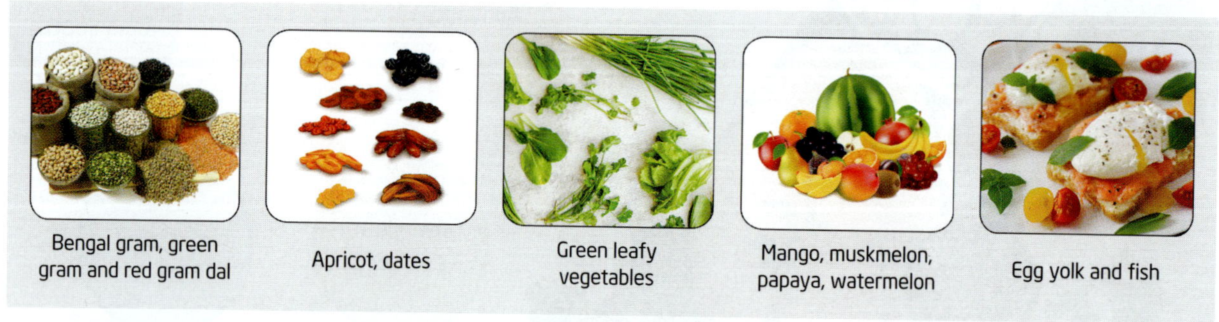

| Bengal gram, green gram and red gram dal | Apricot, dates | Green leafy vegetables | Mango, muskmelon, papaya, watermelon | Egg yolk and fish |

Functions of Vitamin A

- Vitamin A plays a critical role for maintaining normal vision.
- Vitamin A deficiencies are a leading cause of preventable severe visual impairment and blindness.
- Vitamin A helps to improve immunity.
- Adequate amounts of vitamin A in the diet are essential for reproductive health and the healthy development of babies during pregnancy.

* Vitamin A is a fat-soluble vitamin: so eat ghee or oil in sufficient quantity.
* Carrot is a good source of vitamin A: but its absorption increases only when it is cooked in a little fat (not overcook) rather raw.
* Carrot skin has more beta carotene.
* Fruits are a rich source of vitamin A.
* Vitamin A deficiency may increase your risk of developing acne, so if you really don't want acne, try drinking one glass of steamed carrot juice with mint with ½ teaspoon ghee or nuts.
* Excessive consumption of pro- vitamin A may give you nausea, dizziness or headache.

Vitamin D

It is the collective name for cholecalciferol (vitamin D3) and ergocalciferol (vitamin D2). These are precursors of hormones with an important role to play in regulation of the metabolism of calcium and phosphates. Vitamin D is linked with onset of various diseases, so ensure Vitamin D intake.

Vitamin D plays a pivotal role in bone mineral content (BMC) accretion. Suboptimal vitamin D deficiencies contribute to an increased fracture risk.

Though vitamin D requirements range between 400 and 800 IU/day, not all children achieve this. To encourage adequate vitamin D consumption, strategies such as supplementation, sun bath, food labeling and fortification are currently being investigated.

Sources of Vitamin D

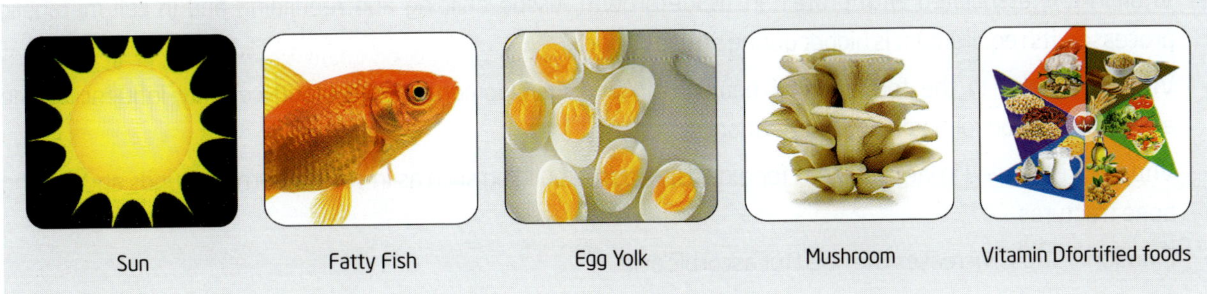

| Sun | Fatty Fish | Egg Yolk | Mushroom | Vitamin Dfortified foods |

Functions of Vitamin D

* Vitamin D increases the muscle strength.
* Vitamin D deficiencies cause low bone density leading to osteoporosis.

Suggestion Box

* If your skin is light, then take 15-20 min sun bath and if your skin is dark then take 30 min sun bath.
* Use soft cotton mulmul cloth while taking sun bath.
* Avoid excessive sun bath, as it has been linked with causing skin disease.

Vitamin C

- It is a water soluble vitamin. Vitamin C is also known as ascorbic acid and ascorbate. It is used to prevent and treat scurvy.
- It is an important vitamin required for the absorption of iron.
- The recommended dietary allowance (RDA) for Vitamin C is 40 mg / day for men, women, children and adolescents.

Sources of Vitamin C

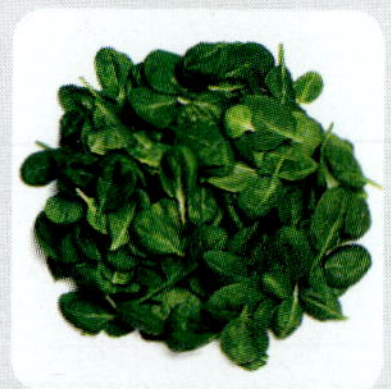

Green leafy vegetables e.g. spinach, amaranth, radish, drumstick leaves, green chilies, green mango, bitter gourd.

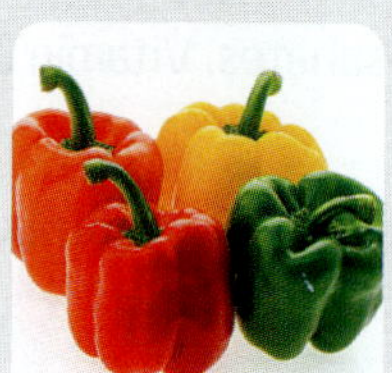

Capsicum/ bell pepper, tomatoes, cabbage.

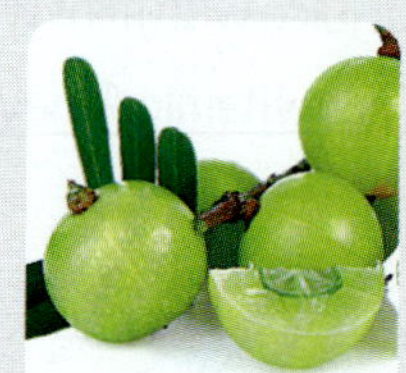

Guava, amla, kiwi.

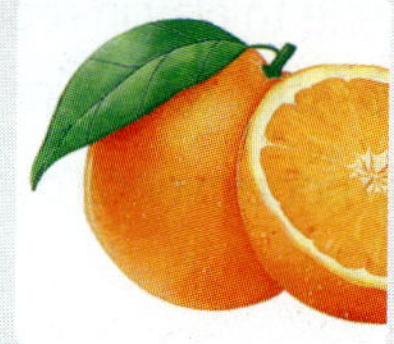

Oranges, lemon, sweet lime, strawberries, all berries and all citrus fruits.

Functions of Vitamin C

- Vitamin C is required to build and maintain bone matrix, cartilage, tooth, collagen and connective tissues.
- Vitamin C is associated with protein in tissue growth, tissue building and rebuilding and in cell metabolic processes, its requirement is higher during stress period.
- Vitamin C helps in the formation of hemoglobin and development of red blood cells by influencing the absorption of iron for hemoglobin formation.
- Vitamin C is needed in large amount for extensive tissue building such as in severe burns, wounds and healing bone fractures.
- Emotional stress increases the need for ascorbic acid.
- Periods such as pregnancy, infancy, and childhood demand more ascorbic acid.
- Deficiency symptoms include bleeding gums, frequent bruising and infections, poor wound healing, anemia and scurvy.

Suggestion Box

- If you do more physical exercise or perspire more than usual, drink orange, sweet lime juice or lemon sharbat.
- Eat seasonal fruit like amla (amla candy, murabba or supari- fresh is a better option). berries, strawberries.
- Simply consuming 100mg of vitamin C may improve iron absorption by 67% so if you have low iron level then add khajur chutney (add some lemon + tamarind + dates) or tomato, beet and spinach juice, in paratha or salad add some seeds like til (sesame seeds).

Vitamin B Complex

B vitamins are a class of water-soluble vitamins that play important roles in cell metabolism. Though these vitamins share similar names, they are chemically distinct compounds that often co-exist in the same foods.

List of Vitamin B

In general, dietary supplements all eight are referred to as a vitamin B complex. Individual B vitamin supplements are referred to by the specific number or name of each vitamin: B1 = thiamine, B2 = riboflavin, B3 = niacin, etc. Some are better known by name than number: niacin, pantothenic acid, biotin and folate.

B Number	Name
Vitamin B1	Thiamine
Vitamin B2	Riboflavin
Vitamin B3	Niacin (Nicotinic Acid) Nicotinamide, Nicotinamide Riboside
Vitamin B5	Pantothenic Acid
Vitamin B6	Pyridoxine, Pyridoxal Pyridoxamine
Vitamin B7	Biotin
Vitamin B8	Folate
Vitamin B12	Various cobalamins; Commonly Cyanocobalamin or Methylcobalamin in vitamin supplements

Sources of Vitamin B

- B vitamins are found in highest abundance in meat.
- They are also found in small quantities in whole unprocessed carbohydrate-based foods.
- Good sources for vitamins B include legumes (pulses or beans), chili peppers, nutritional yeast , eggs, liver and kidneys chicken and red meat, fish, shellfish such as oysters.
- Dark green vegetables such as spinach and vegetables such as beets, avocados, and potatoes are also an excellent source.
- Whole grains and cereals.
- Beans, such as kidney beans, black beans, and chickpeas.
- Nuts and seeds.
- Fruits such as citrus, banana, and watermelon.
- Soya milk.
- Wheat germ.

Deficiencies of Vitamin B

Several named vitamin deficiency diseases may result from the lack of sufficient B vitamins. Deficiencies of other B vitamins result in symptoms that are not part of a named deficiency disease.

B Number	Name	Deficiency effect
Vitamin B1	Thiamine	Deficiency causes beriberi (nervous system includes weight loss, emotional disturbances), weakness and pain in the limbs, periods of irregular heartbeat, and swelling of body. Heart failure and death may occur in advanced cases.
Vitamin B2	Riboflavin	Riboflavin deficiency causes cracks in the lips, high sensitivity to sunlight, inflammation of the tongue, sore throat
Vitamin B3	Niacin	Deficiency, along with a deficiency of tryptophan, causes pellagra. Symptoms include. 4 D – 1D dermatitis, weakness, mental confusion, 2D diarrhea. 3D dementia and 4D death
Vitamin B5	Pantothenic acid	Deficiency can result in acne although it is uncommon.
Vitamin B6	Pyridoxine, Pyridoxal, Pyridoxamine	Vitamin B6 deficiency causes eruptions, pink eye and neurological symptoms (e.g. epilepsy).
Vitamin B7	Biotin	Deficiency leads to decreased nail and hair growth
Vitamin B9	Folic acide	Deficiency results in anemia. Deficiency in pregnant women can lead to birth defects.
Vitamin B12	Cobalamin	Deficiency results in anemia, memory loss and, neurological disorders other cognitive deficits.

Suggestion Box

- Niacin is important for healthy skin.
- Biotin is good for hair and skin.
- Vitamin B6 good for brain development.
- If you get irritated which is a typical symptom in teenagers, then have a good amount of Vitamin B6 because it helps to release serotonin which regulates moods.
- Vitamin B6 also helps if girls have cramps during menstrual cycle.

Minerals

Minerals constitute three to four percent of the total body weight.

They help build tissues and regulate body fluids in various body functions.

Much like the vitamins, minerals are also required in small quantities.

They should be supplied daily as they get excreted through the kidney, the bowel and the skin.

Examples of Minerals are

Calcium, phosphorus, potassium, sodium, iodine, iron, copper, molybdenum, Sulphur, chlorine, magnesium, manganese etc.

Minerals are classified into three groups

A. **Major minerals**

   These are required in large quantity. E.g.: Calcium

B. **Minor minerals**

   These are required in small quantity. E.g.: Iron, Magnesium.

C. **Trace elements**

   They are required in extremely small quantity like few micrograms.

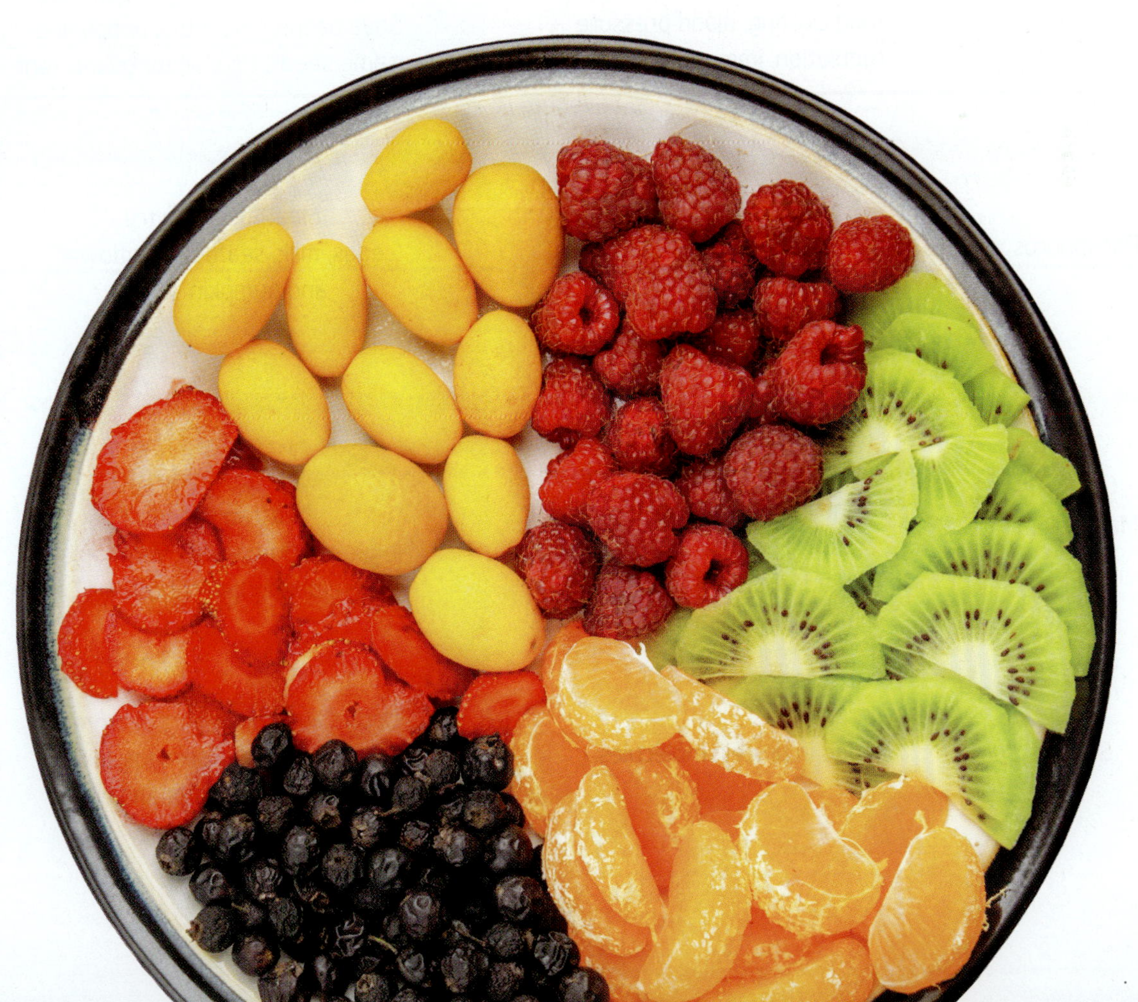

Mineral	Function	Sources
Sodium	To control blood pressure, Needed for proper fluid balance, nerve transmission, and muscle contraction.	Table salt, soya sauce; high in processed foods; breads, pizza, unprocessed meats, tacos, chips, kurkure, (intake of sodium should be in moderate amount).
Chloride	It helps keep fluid inside and outside of cells in balance, it maintains stomach acid and blood volume.	Table salt, soya sauce; large amounts in processed foods; meats and breads.
Potassium	Needed for proper fluid balance, nerve functions, and muscle contraction.	Meats, potatoes, spinach, sweet potatoes, mushrooms, bananas, oranges, watermelons, coconut water, white beans, dried apricots, beetroots, pomegranates.
Calcium	Building strong bones and teeth; helps muscles relax and contract; important in nerve function, blood clotting, blood pressure regulation, immune system.	Milk and milk products; Green leafy vegetables – such as broccoli, cabbage and okra, but not spinach. Soya beans, tofu, nuts, poppy and sesame seeds, fish, white beans, ragi.
Phosphorus	Formation of bones and teeth; needed for body to make protein for the growth, maintenance and repair found in every cell; part of the system that maintain acid-base balance.	Meat, fish, poultry, eggs, milk, seafood, sunflower and pumpkin seeds.
Magnesium	Regulate blood pressure, need magnesium to make antioxidant Found in bones; needed for making protein, muscle contraction, nerve transmission, immune system health.	Avocado, fatty fish, Nuts and seeds; legumes; green leafy vegetables; seafood; dark chocolate.
Sulfur	Found in protein molecules.	Occurs in foods as part of protein: meats, poultry, fish, eggs, milk, legumes, onion, garlic and nuts.

Trace Minerals

Mineral	Function	Sources
Iron	Part of a molecule (hemoglobin) found in red blood cells that carries oxygen in the body; needed for energy metabolism	Organ meats; red meats; fish; poultry; shellfish; egg yolks; legumes; beans and peas, nuts and seeds, pumpkin, sesame seeds, flaxseeds, prunes, amaranth, soyabean , dark green leafy vegetables ; iron-enriched breads and cereals; and fortified cereals
Zinc	Part of many enzymes; needed for making protein and genetic material; has a function in taste perception, wound healing, normal fetal development, production of sperm, normal growth and sexual maturation, immune system health, good for skin and hair	Meats, fish, poultry, legumes – chick peas, seeds-pumpkin and sesame, nuts - peanuts , cashewnuts and almonds, whole grains, green leafy vegetables and potatoes , mustard seeds, sesame seeds
Iodine	Found in thyroid hormone, which helps regulate growth, development, and metabolism	Seafood, fish, foods grown in iodine-rich soil, iodized salt, fortified bread, dairy products
Selenium	Selenium helps to make antioxidant enzymes. These play a role in preventing cell damage	Meats, seafood, grains, whole grains, nuts and seeds, eggs, fish
Copper	Works with iron; needed for iron metabolism, helps to increase immune system	Legumes, nuts and seeds, whole grains, organ meats, drinking water
Manganese	It is involved in amino acids, cholesterol, glucose and carbohydrate Metabolism	Nuts, soybeans, leafy vegetables, black pepper
Fluoride	Involved in formation of bones and teeth; helps prevent tooth decay	Drinking water, fish
Chromium	It aids in insulin to regulate blood sugar (glucose) levels, important in the breakdown of fats and carbohydrates	Unrefined foods, broccoli, grapes, apple, bananas, potatoes, yeast, whole grains, nuts, cheese, seafood, non-vegetarian food
Molybdenum	Helps break down Proteins	Legumes; breads and grains; leafy greens; leafy, green vegetables; milk; liver

Calcium

Calcium is an essential nutrient that is necessary for many functions in human health. Calcium is the most abundant mineral in the body with 99% found in teeth and bone.

Calcium metabolism involves other nutrients including proteins, vitamin D, and phosphorus. Bone formation and maintenance is a lifelong process. Early attention to strong bones in childhood and adulthood will provide more stable bone mass during the aging years.

Research has shown that adequate calcium intake can reduce the risk of fractures, osteoporosis, and diabetes in some populations.

It is important to remember that it is difficult if not impossible to discuss calcium alone. Calcium metabolism is a collaborative effort between calcium, phosphorus, vitamin D, and proteins. Just like a musical orchestra, all of these nutrients are needed to create the end product whether it is a beautiful song or a perfect bone matrix.

Sources of Calcium

- Milk and milk products.
- Green leafy vegetables – such as Fenugreek leaves, betel leaves
- Drumsticks, radish leaves, amaranth and curry leaves, broccoli, cabbage, Okra (BHINDI), and soya beans (tofu, soya milk).
- Almonds, raisins and figs.
- Oil seeds such as gingelly, poppy seeds, ajwain, coriander seeds, mustard, garden cress.
- Egg yolk.
- Legumes such as rajma, horse gram, rajgeera, moth beans. Ragi.
- Fish such as sardines.

Functions of Calcium

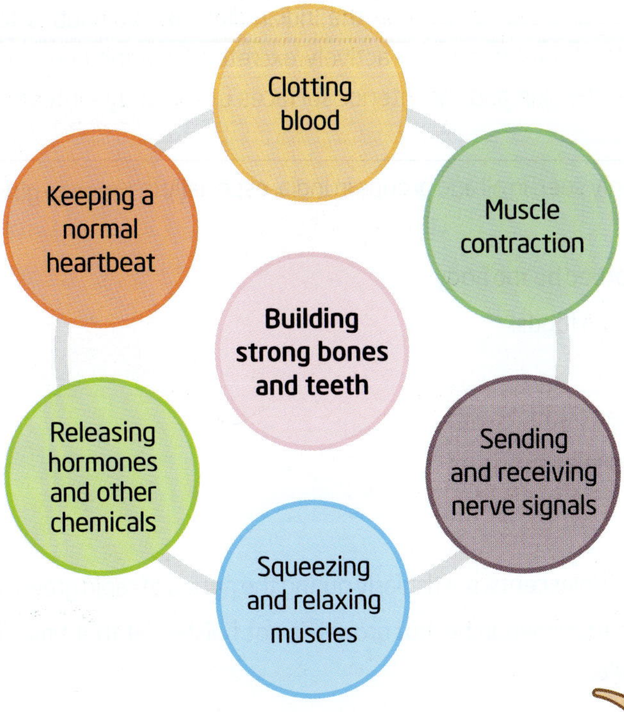

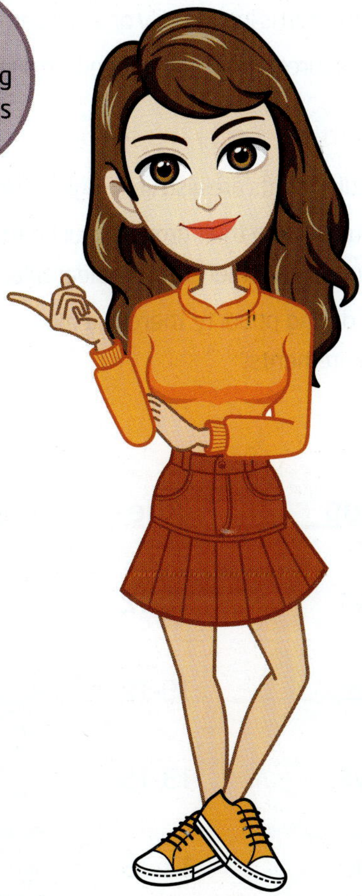

Deficiency of Calcium

It can cause :

- Osteoporosis and osteopenia.
- Fatigue and lethargy.
- Painful menstrual cycle.
- Dental problems.
- Confusion or memory loss.
- Muscle spasm / cramps.
- Numbness and tingling in the hands, feet, and face.
- Depression.
- Weak and brittle nails.
- Frequent fracture of the bones.

Suggestion Box

- Adequate intake of milk and milk products should be ensured.
- Calcium is like a bank balance. More bank balance = more money = more calcium = More healthy bones.
- There are also other good sources than milk like poppy seeds, ragi, and curry leaves, so eat ragi roti or mix ragi flour in your normal wheat flour.
- Eat green chutney with curry leaves and poppy seeds every day.
- Eat almonds and green leafy vegetables.

Iron

Though Iron is an essential nutrient, it is generally deficient in the Indian diet. Its main job is to carry oxygen throughout your body as a part of red blood cells. Iron is not actively excreted from the body in urine or in the intestines. Iron is only lost with cells from the skin and the interior surfaces of the body - intestines and urinary tract.

Deficiency of Iron called Anemia is commonly seen in all age groups in India, especially in teenage girls.

Heme Iron :

- Heme iron is more easily used and absorbed by the body.
- It can be sourced from the non-vegetarian foods.

Non-Heme Iron

- Non-heme iron is less readily or absorbed by our bodies.
- It can be sourced from grains, seeds, fruits and veggies.

Recommended Daily Allowances

- Iron requirements are also very high in adolescents, particularly during the period of rapid growth.
- Girls usually have their growth spurt before menarche, but growth is not finished at that time. Their total iron requirements are therefore considerable.
- In boys during puberty there is a marked increase in hemoglobin mass and concentration, further increasing iron requirements.

Group	Age	Iron – mg/day
Boys	10-12	21
Girls	10-12	27
Boys	13-15	32
Girls	13-15	27

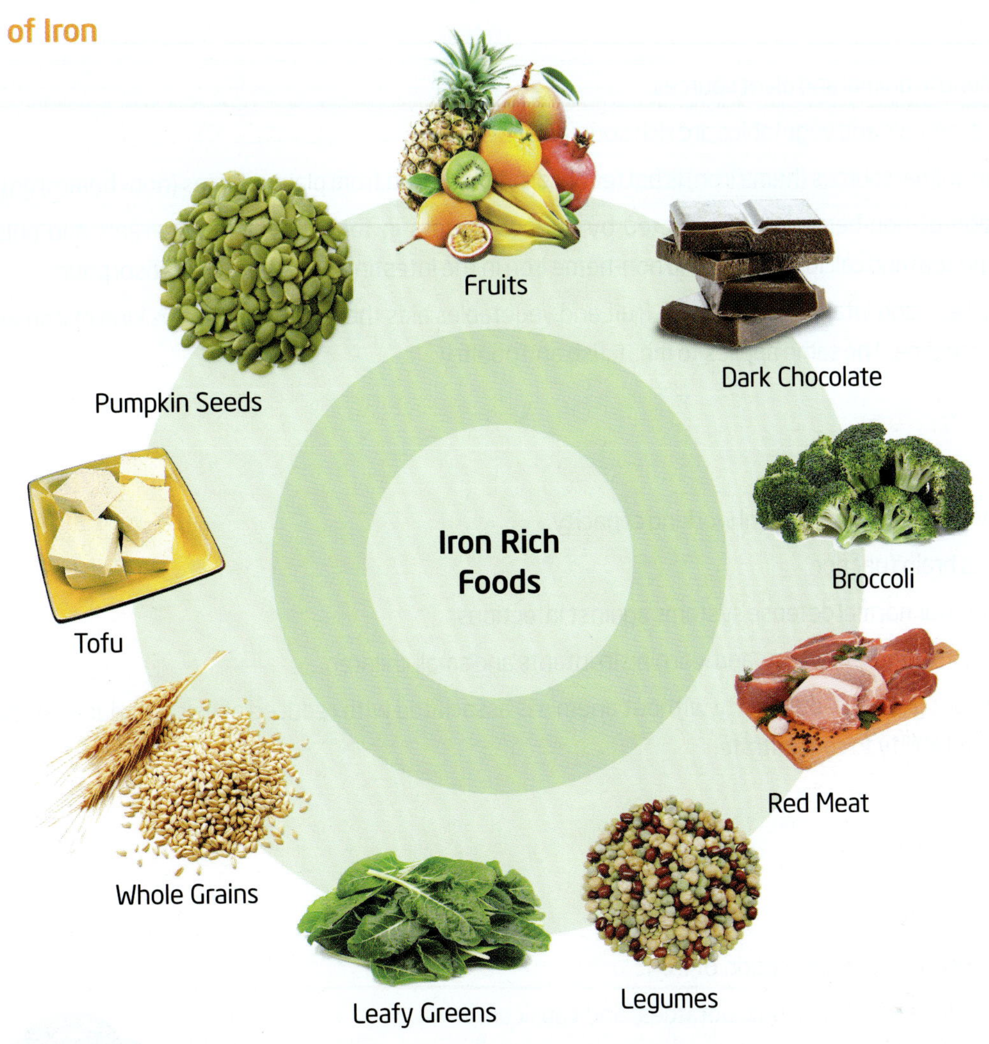

Vitamin C increases effect of iron absorption

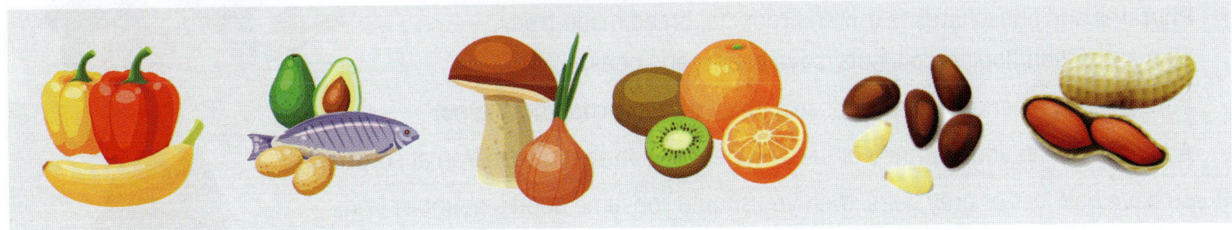

Functions of Iron

- Hemoglobin's primary role is to transport oxygen from the lungs to the body tissues.

- Iron is necessary for immune cells proliferation and maturation, particularly of lymphocytes.

- It keeps you active and energetic.

- Iron boosts our immunity.

Sources

- Iron is found in animal and plant sources.
- Red meat, cereals and vegetables are rich sources.
- Iron from animal sources (heme iron) is better absorbed than iron from plant sources (non- heme iron).
- Absorption of non-heme iron is affected by various factors in food. Phytate (in cereals and pulses), fiber, tannins (in tea) and calcium can all bind non-heme iron in the intestine, which reduces absorption.
- On the other hand vitamin C, present in fruit and vegetables aids the absorption of this kind of iron when eaten at the same time. The same applies to meat, fish and poultry.

Deficiency of Iron

Leads to :

- Significant reduction in physical working capacity.
- Decreases brain function.
- Diminishes our normal defense systems against infections.
- Effects on attention, memory, and learning in infants and small children.
- In adolescent girls, iron-deficiency without anemia is associated with reduced physical endurance and changes in mood and ability to concentrate.

Suggestion Box

Enhancing Factors :

These Food increase the absorption of iron :

- Ascorbic acid (e.g., Citrus fruits, potatoes, and capsicum).
- Meat chicken fish and other seafood.
- High protein food.

Inhibiting Factors :

These factors interfere with the absorption of iron so you should avoid these foods :

- Phytates and phosphates (e.g. bran products, bread made from high extraction flour, cocoa, nuts, soya beans, and peas).
- Iron – binding phenolic compounds (e.g. tea, coffee, cocoa, chocolates)
- Adding lemon in your chutney or juices is best option to increase iron absorption.

If you have hair loss or grey hairs, then you should consume good amount of iron.

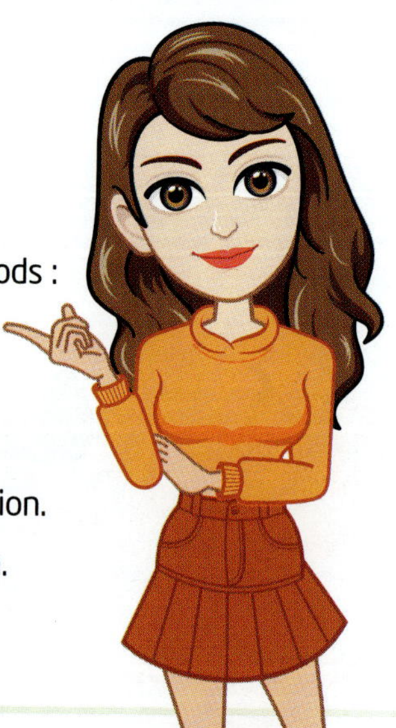

Electrolyte Balance

Kids, what are "Electrolytes"?

Sodium, potassium, chloride and bicarbonate are blood electrolytes. They help regulate nerve and muscle function and maintain acid-base balance as well as water balance.

Having these electrolytes in the right concentration is called electrolyte balance. It is important for maintaining fluid balance among the various compartments of our body.

Any idea why do we need to talk about "Electrolyte Balance"?

That is because, we are super active, and we tend to lose more electrolytes through loss of fluid during these activities. And an imbalance in electrolytes can result in fatigue, lethargy, nausea, vomiting, abdominal cramps and muscle weakness.

Causes of Electrolyte Imbalance

- Severe diarrhea.
- Sweating.
- Fluid loss from heavy exercise or physical activity.

Suggestion Box

- Stay hydrated during your exercise.
- Stay hydrated if you are suffering from vomiting, diarrhea and sweating.
- Athletes need more electrolyte balance; so they should drink electrolyte fluid.
- Drink when you are thirsty, Don't be lazy!

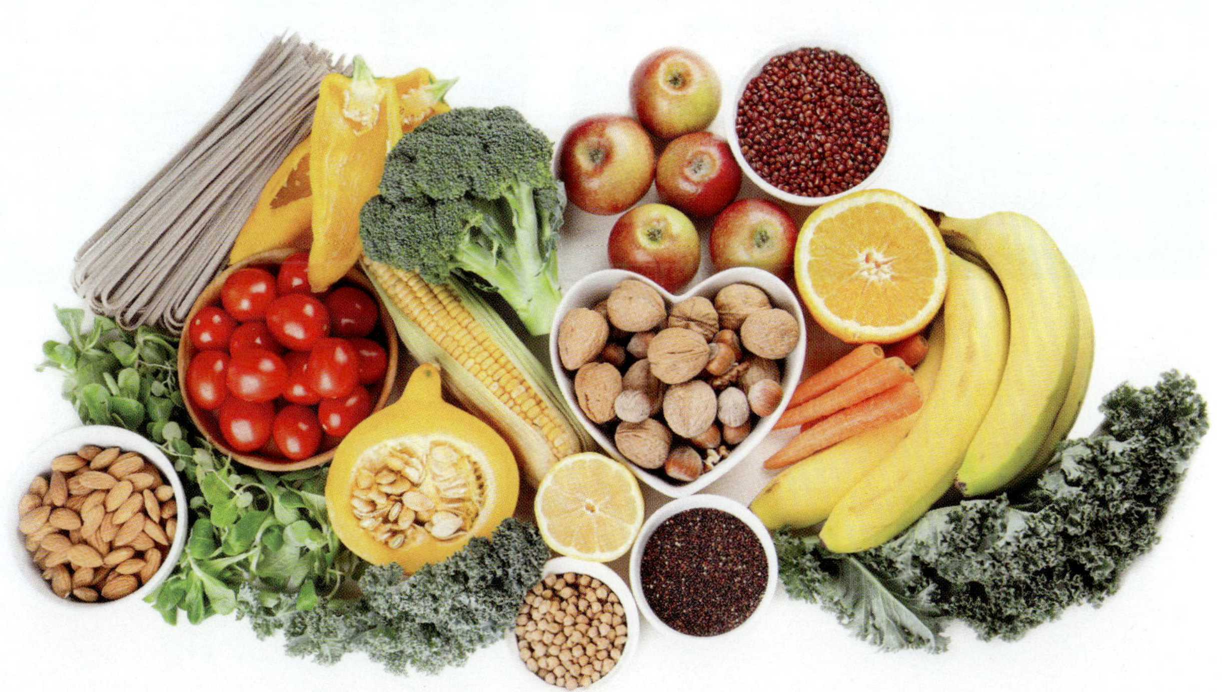

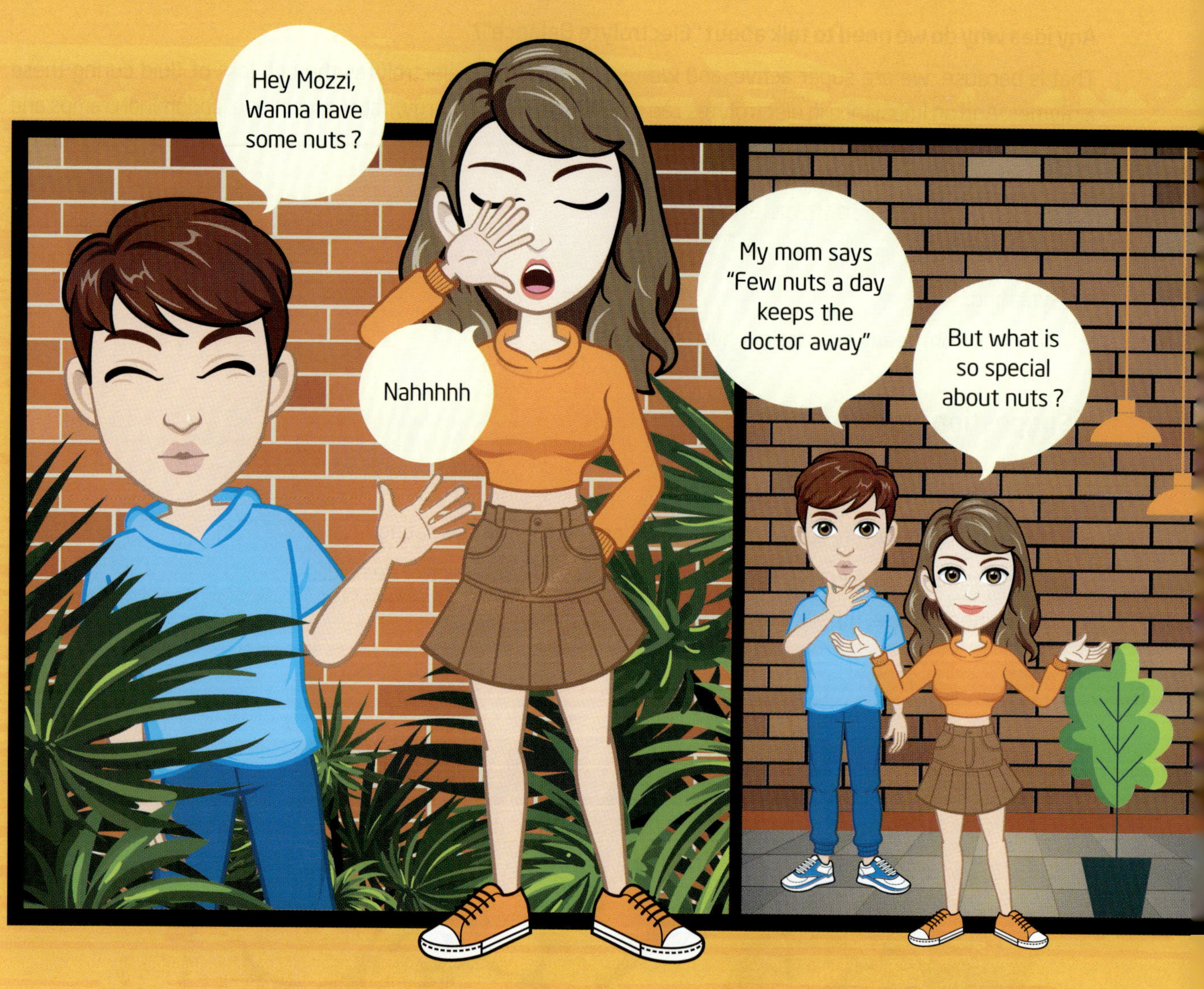

Hey Mozzi, Wanna have some nuts ?
Nahhhhh
My mom says "Few nuts a day keeps the doctor away"
But what is so special about nuts ?

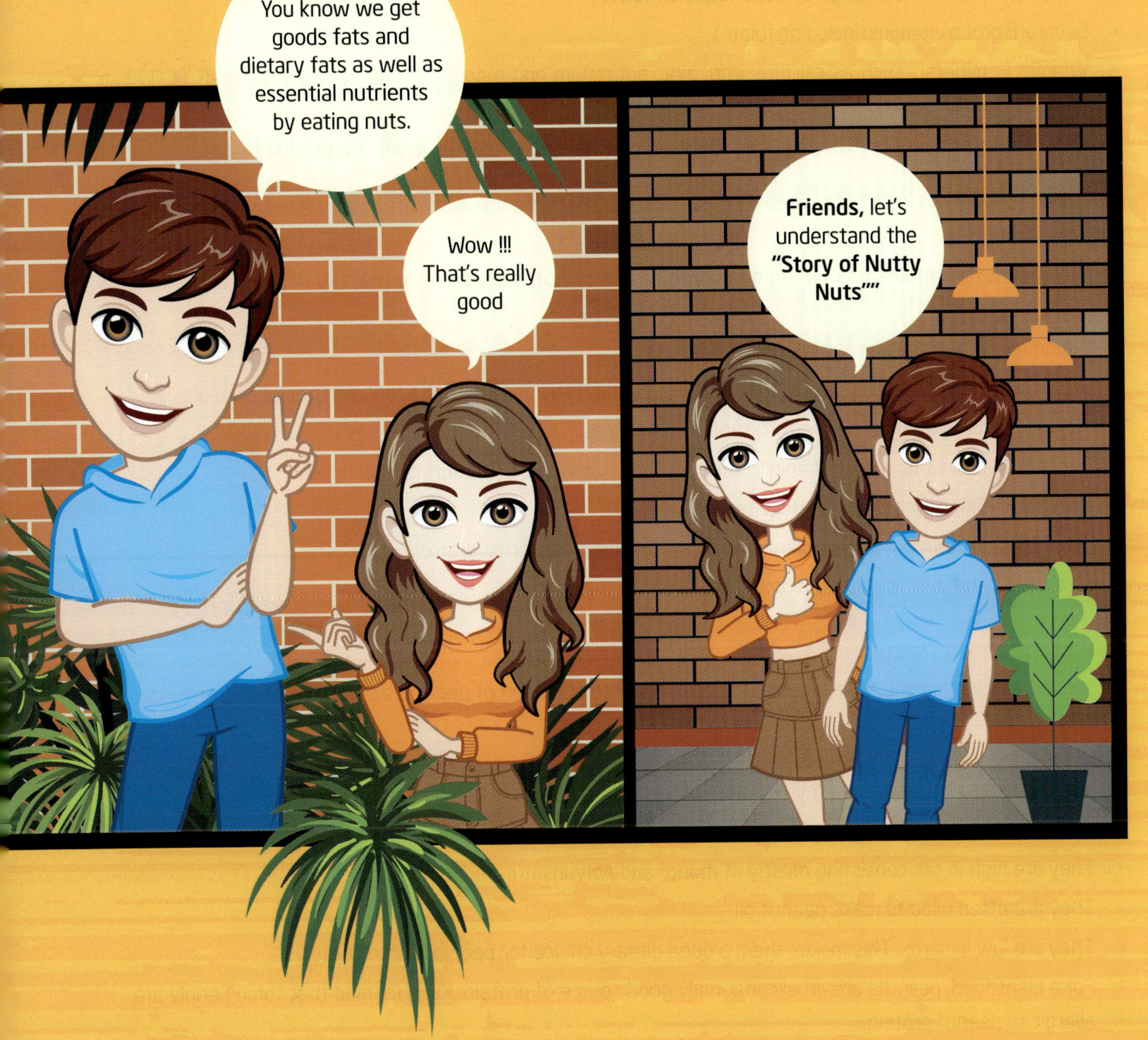

6. Story of Nutty Nuts

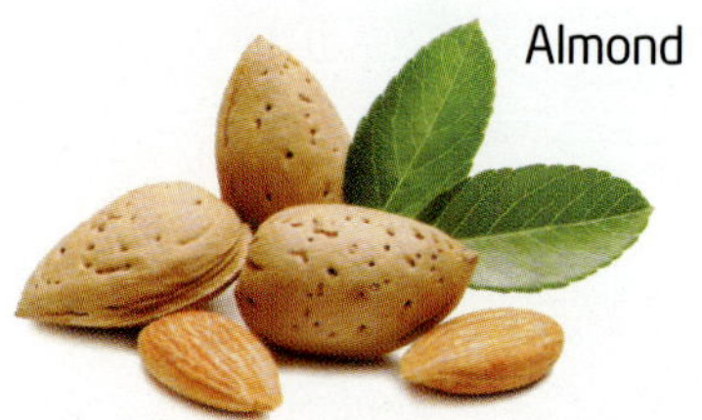

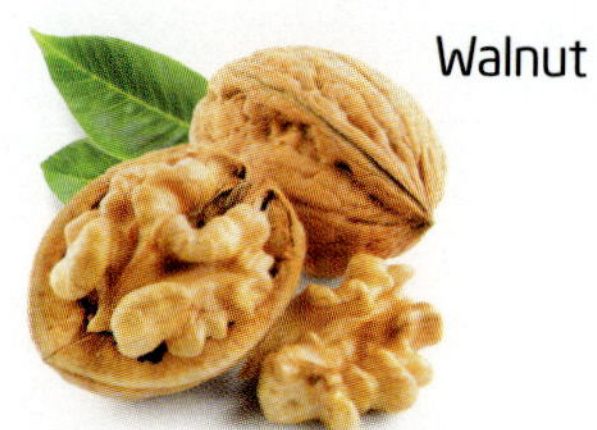

Kids, the easiest way to get good fats as well as dietary fiber is by eating nuts.

Nuts also provide a wide range of essential nutrients –

- Several B group vitamins (including folate).
- Vitamin E, minerals such as calcium, iron, zinc, potassium and magnesium, antioxidant minerals (selenium, manganese and copper).
- Other phytochemicals such as antioxidant compounds (flavonoids and resveratrol) and plant sterols.

Nuts are naturally low in sodium, contain potassium and most contain some carbohydrate in the form of natural sugars.

Each nut variety contains its own unique combination of nutrients and is generally rich in a few nutrients such as:

- Almonds - Protein, calcium and vitamin E.
- Brazil nuts - Fiber and selenium. Just two Brazil nuts a day provides 100% RDI for selenium for an adult.
- Cashews-Non - heme (plant based) iron and a low GI rating.
- Chestnuts - Low GI, fiber and vitamin C (although much vitamin C is lost during cooking).
- Hazelnuts - Fiber, potassium, folate, vitamin E.
- Pistachios - Protein, potassium, plant sterols and the antioxidant resveratrol.
- Walnuts - Alpha linoleic acid: plant omega 3 and antioxidants.

Let's talk about Peanuts !

Although peanut is technically a legume, the nutritional composition of peanut is close to that of tree nuts.

Peanuts

- Peanuts are packed with healthy fats and high-quality protein.
- They're also fairly high in calories.
- They are high in fat, consisting mostly of mono- and polyunsaturated fatty acids.
- They are often used to make peanut oil.
- They are low in carbs. This makes them a good dietary choice for people with diabetes.
- For a plant food, peanuts are an exceptionally good source of protein. Keep in mind that some people are allergic to peanut protein.
- They are an excellent source of many vitamins and minerals. These include biotin, copper, niacin, folate, manganese, vitamin E, thiamine, phosphorus, and magnesium.
- They contain various plant compounds. These include antioxidants, such as coumaric acid and resveratrol, as well as anti-nutrients like phytic acid.

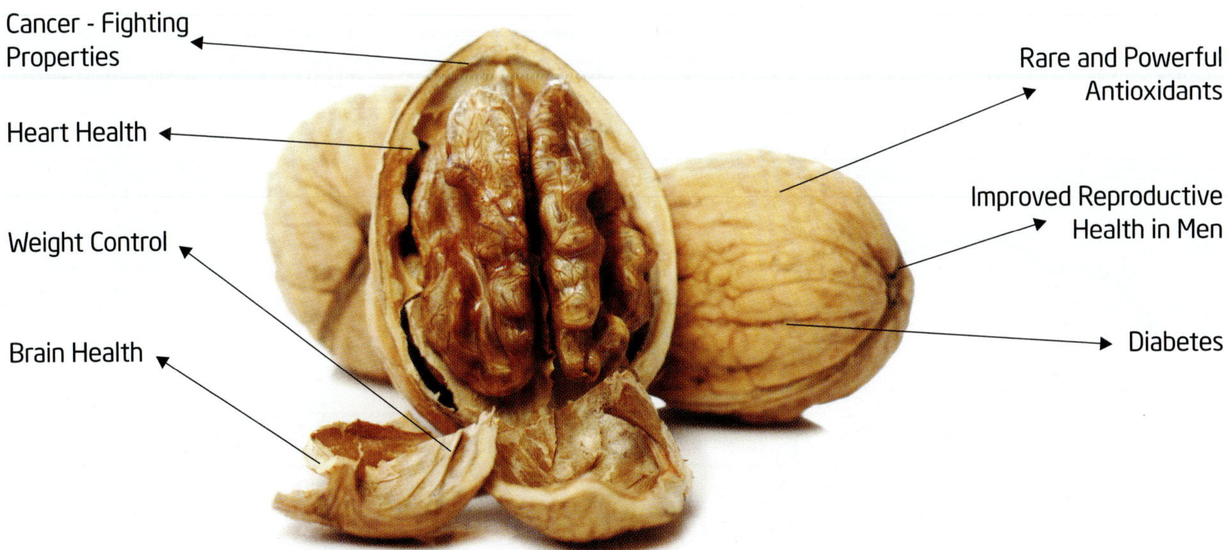

Know Your Nuts

Walnuts
High in omega 3 fatty acids
Benefits : Fights heart disease, cancer, diabetes, high blood pressure

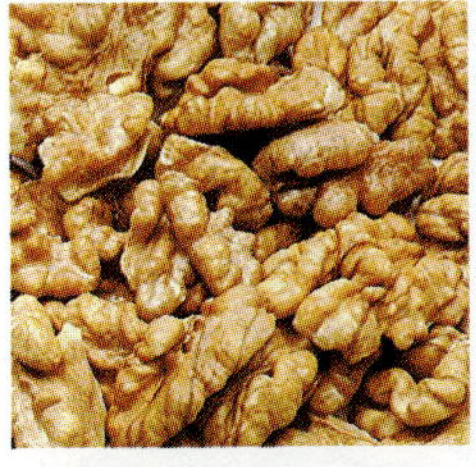

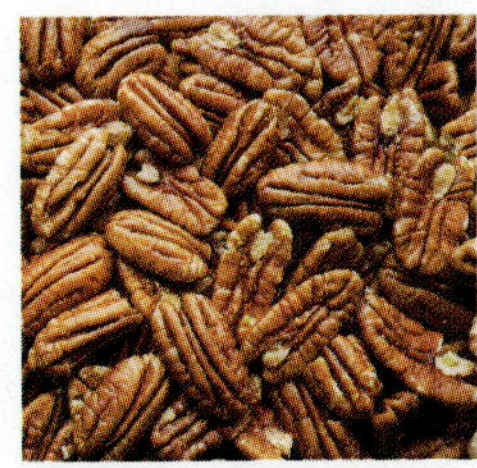

Pecans
Vitamin A&E, Zinc
Benefits :
Lowers cholesterols

Almonds
High in protein, zinc and calcium
Benefits :
Reduces bad cholesterol

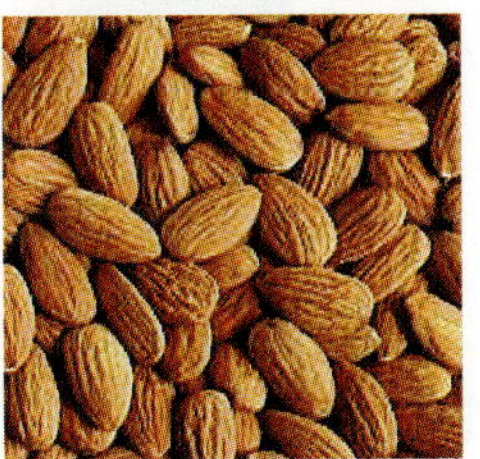

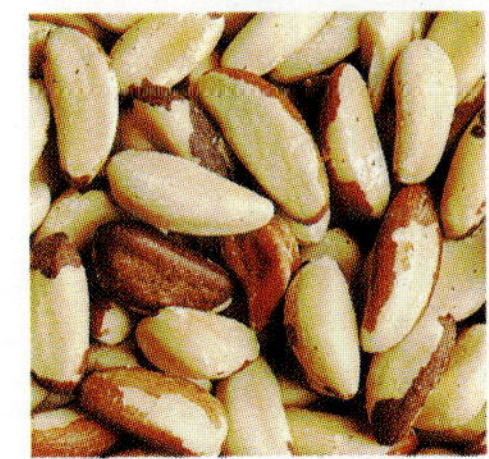

Brazil Nuts
Antioxidant, high in minerals
Benefits :
Improves mental health

Cashew Nuts
Protein and Fiber
Benefits : Heart health, aid in weight loss

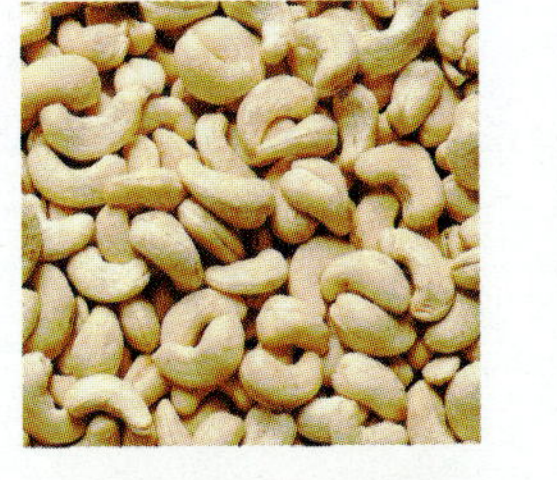

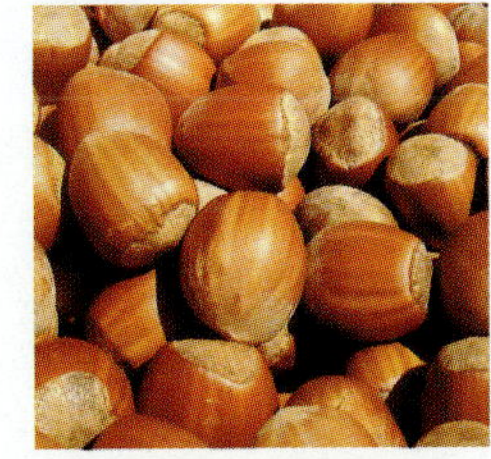

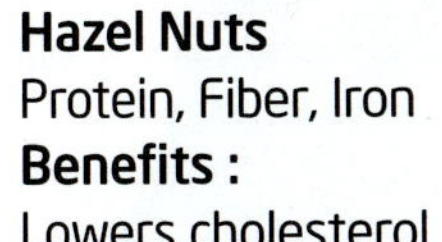

Hazel Nuts
Protein, Fiber, Iron
Benefits :
Lowers cholesterol

Pine Nuts
Vitamin A,C & D
Befefits :
Strengthens immunity

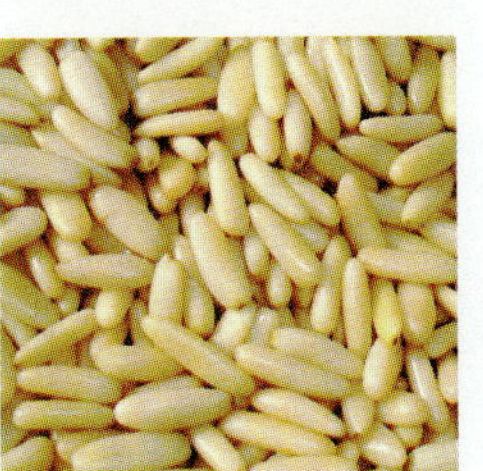

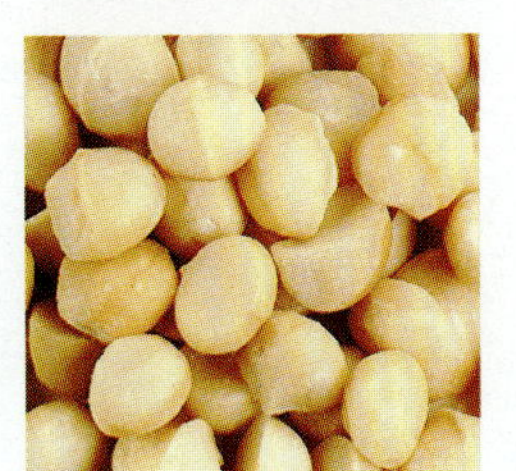

Macadamia Nuts
Rich in omega 3, Vitamin A
Benefits :
Increases metabolism

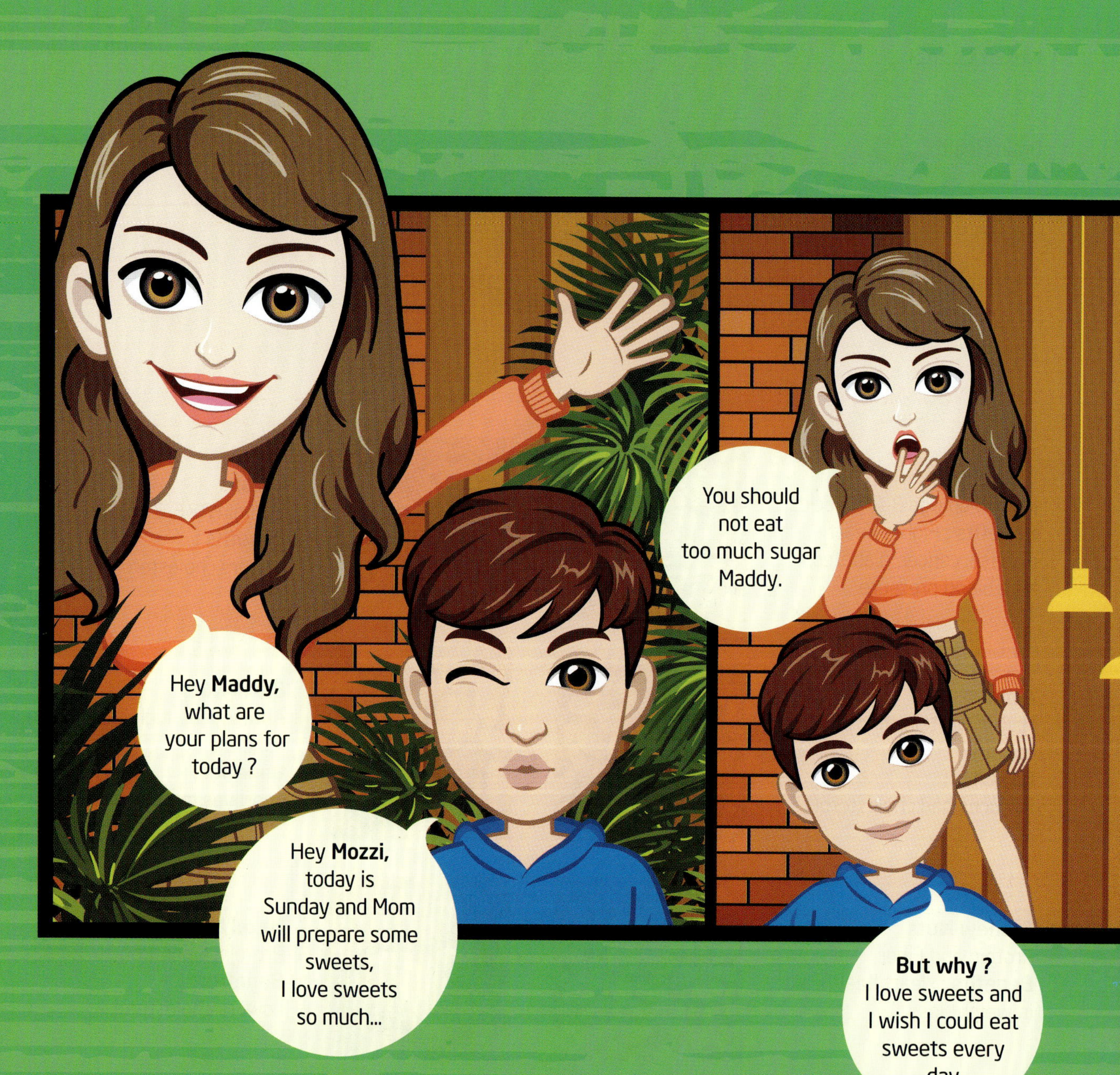

Hey Maddy, what are your plans for today ?
Hey Mozzi, today is Sunday and Mom will prepare some sweets, I love sweets so much...
You should not eat too much sugar Maddy.
But why ? I love sweets and I wish I could eat sweets every day

It is found in all food in some form or the other. When it comes to nutrition, the real corona is Sugar.
Hmm...
Friends, let's understand the bitter story of "Sugar"

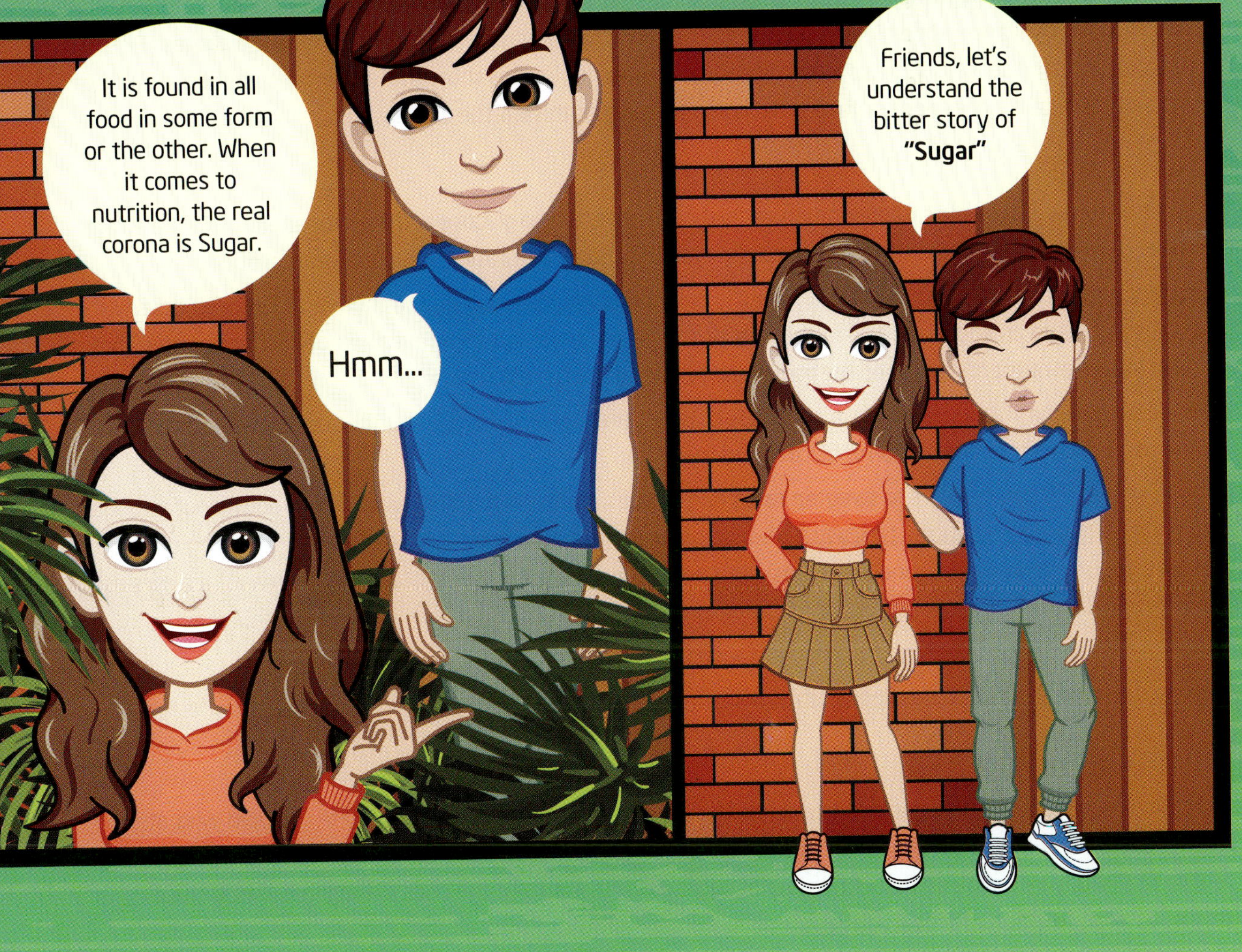

7. Sugar

Hey Kids, you've all heard about corona, right? The virus impacted our health during the pendemic.

When it comes to nutrition, the real corona is Sugar.

It is found in all food in some form or the other.

In India, we have a close relationship to sugar.

You will observe, we start our day with prasad. We tend to have desserts on multiple days in a week, we have different variety of sweets on birthdays, marriages, functions festivals etc. India produces around 32 million tons of sugar and consumes 25 million tons.

Increasing trend of per capita sugar consumption assumes significance in view of the high tendency for Indians to develop insulin resistance, abdominal adiposity, obesity and the increasing "epidemic" of type 2 diabetes (T2DM) and cardiovascular diseases. In this context, dietary guidelines for Indians show that sugar consumption should be less than 10% of total daily energy intake, but it is suggested that this limit be decreased.

What is Sugar?

Sugar, in all forms, is a simple carbohydrate that the body converts into glucose and uses for energy. But the effect on the body and your overall health depends on the type of sugar you're eating, either natural or refined.

Natural sugars are found in fruits as fructose and in dairy products, such as milk and cheese, as lactose. Foods with natural sugar have an important role in the diet of cancer patients and for prevention of cancer because they provide essential nutrients that keep the body healthy and helps prevent disease.

Refined sugar comes from sugar cane or sugar beets, which are processed to extract the sugar. It is typically found as sucrose, which is the combination of glucose and fructose.

We use white and brown sugars to sweeten cakes and cookies, coffee, cereal and even fruits. Food manufacturers add chemically produced sugar, typically high-fructose corn syrup, to foods and beverages, including crackers, flavored yogurt, tomato sauce and salad dressing. Low-fat foods are the worst offenders, as manufacturers use sugar to add flavor. Most of the processed foods we eat add calories and sugar with little nutritional value.

In contrast, fruits and unsweetened milk have vitamins and minerals.

Milk also has protein and fruit has fiber, both of which make you feel full for a longer time.

Bitter truth about sugar:

According to a study published in the Journal of the American Medical Association (JAMA), people who ate the largest amounts of added sugar had the highest blood triglyceride levels and the lowest HDL (good) cholesterol levels. That study also showed that eating lots of sugar more than tripled the odds of having low HDL cholesterol levels, a strong risk factor for heart disease.

What are the substitutes for white sugar?

Sugar = Jaggery = honey, all give the same amount of calories but jaggery & honey are healthier than sugar. They should also be used in limited quantity.

Substitute of sugar

Honey, Stevia , Molasses, Maple Syrup, Jaggery, Gaddi Shakkar, Brown Sugar or Organic Sugar, Fruit Juices and Sugarcane Juice, Dates

Sugar in Different drinks

Drink type	Type of sugar	Average quantity of sugar in teaspoons
Water	No sugar and essential for health and hydration	
Milk (250ml)	Natural sugar	3 teaspoons
Fruit juice 100% natural (250 ml)	Natural sugar - but drinking too much can cause tooth decay	6 teaspoons
Flavored milk	Natural and added sugar - drinking too much can lead to increased weight gain	7 teaspoons
Flavored fruit drink 250ml	Added sugar	6.5 teaspoons
Energy drink 600ml	Added sugar	8.5 teaspoons
Soft drink can 375ml	Added sugar	9 teaspoons
Soft drink (buddy)-600ml	Added sugar	15 teaspoons
Soft drinks 1.25 lit bottle 1250 ml	Highly added sugar	33 teaspoons

Why we should avoid High added sugar drinks ?

Soft drinks & other high sugar drinks such as energy drinks, flavored mineral waters, fruit drinks and sports drinks can contain amounts of sugar in excess of dietary needs. Drinking too many high sugar drinks can contribute to :

- Obesity
- Tooth decay
- Weight gain
- When lots of sugary drinks are consumed on a regular basis, the body can't use all the sugar and turns it into fat. Being overweight can contribute to Heart Disease, diabetes and other chronic diseases.
- High blood sugar levels and increased weight gain can place strain on key organs such as the heart and kidneys.

Other side effects about high sugar diets

Increases acne, Type 2 diabetes, Increases the risk of cancer, Increases risk of depression, Increases PCOD / PCOS problems in girls, leads to fatty liver.

Suggestion Box

- Don't add sugar in your milk and sherbet, instead add Honey, jaggery (in limited quantity)
- Milk protein chocolate powder has sugar, so while adding in your milk add a small amount or avoid it.
- Cakes and pastries are the real monsters, so eat them in limited quantity.
- Sauces and ketchup also have a good amount of hidden sugar, so take it in smaller quantity.
- Avoid jams, ice-creams which are high in refined sugar.

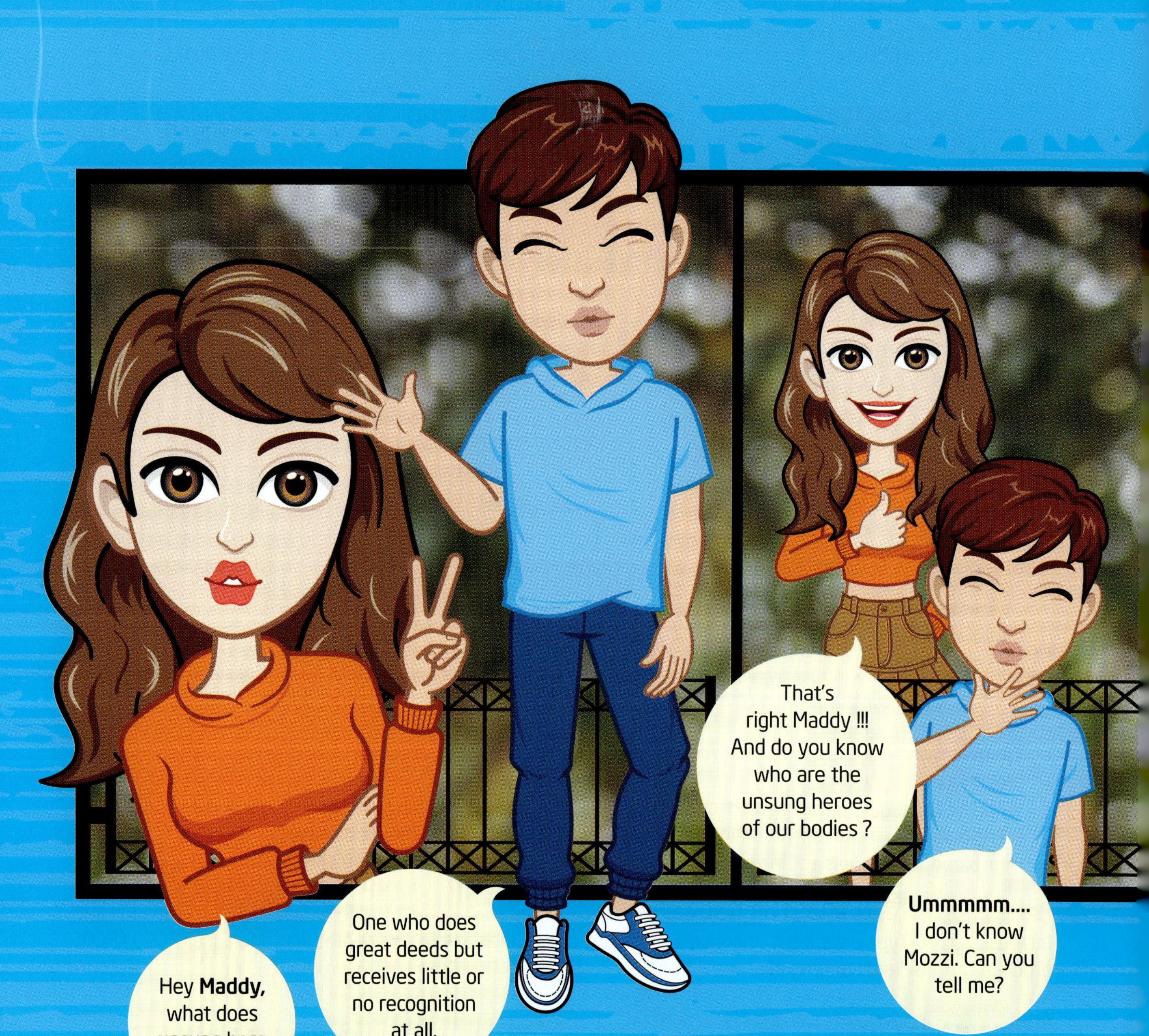

Hey Maddy, what does unsung hero mean?
One who does great deeds but receives little or no recognition at all.
That's right Maddy !!! And do you know who are the unsung heroes of our bodies ?
Ummmmm.... I don't know Mozzi. Can you tell me?

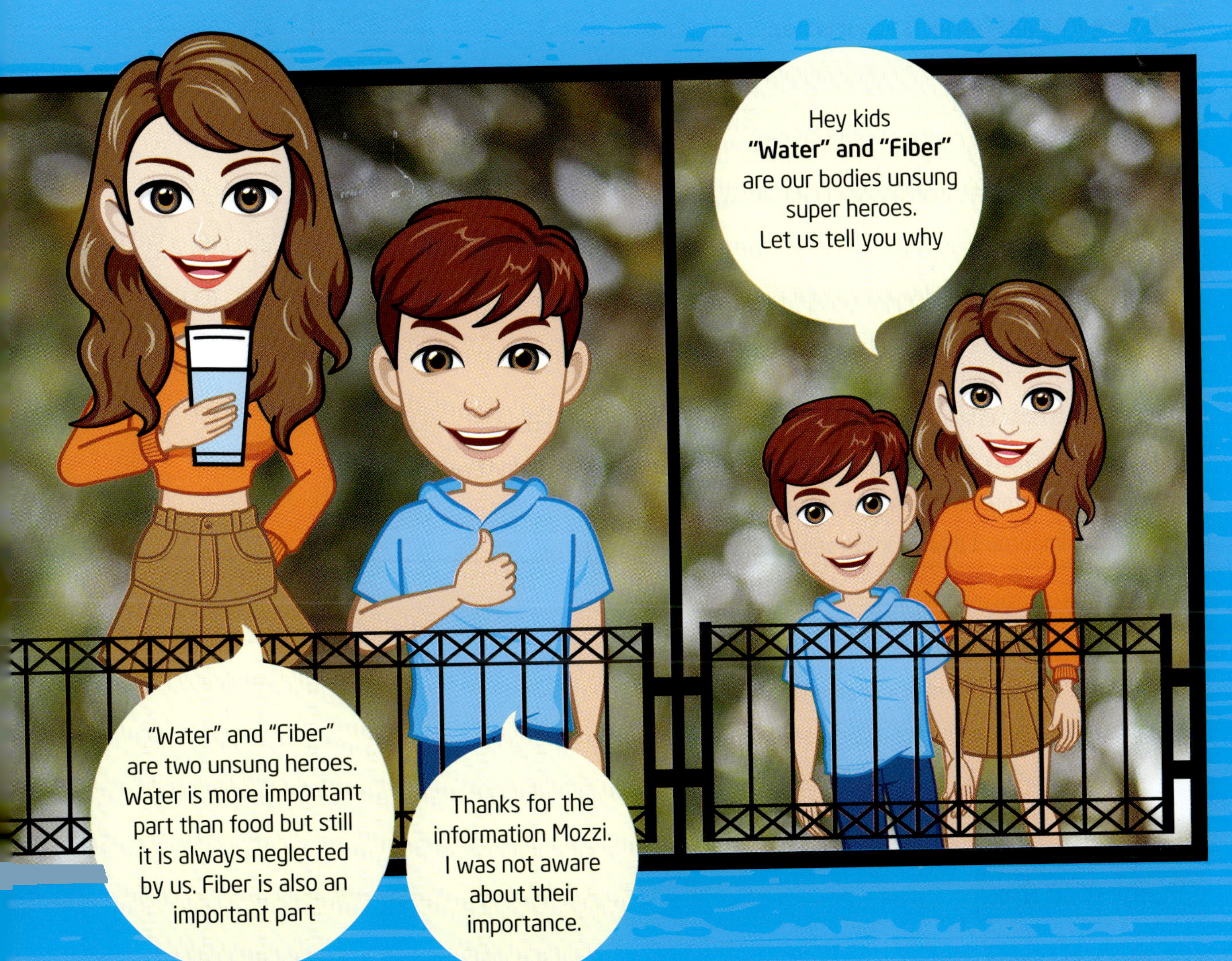

8. Water and Fiber

Nutrients In Water

- Chlorine, Potassium, Phosphorus, Mo.y... ...
- Calcium, Magnesium, Sodium, Potassium.
- Ferrous iron, Copper, Zinc, Manganese.
- Iodine, Chromium.
- Boron, Chromium, Nickel, Silicon, Vanadium

Water

Kids, here are some fun facts about Water:

- Our body contains about 65% to 70% water.
- An infant's body contains more water than an adult.
- A thin person has higher percentage of water than a fat person.
- Men have more water than women in their body.

Functions of Water

- It is found around and in the cells as well as in the organs.
- It maintains our body temperature.
- It maintains electrolyte balance.
- It keeps nutrients in solution form so that nutrients are easily absorbed.
- It acts as vehicle for the waste products which are excreted through the bowel or kidney.
- It lubricates and prevents friction e.g.: saliva.

Water is more important than food but still it is always neglected by us.

Calculate your water intake

- 30 - 50 ml * your ideal body weight if you are more active = 70 ml * your ideal body weight.
- Check your urine and drink water accordingly.
    - a. Transparent urine – no need to increase your water intake.
    - b. Light yellow colour – increase - 500ml.
    - c. Dark yellow Urine – increase 700ml.

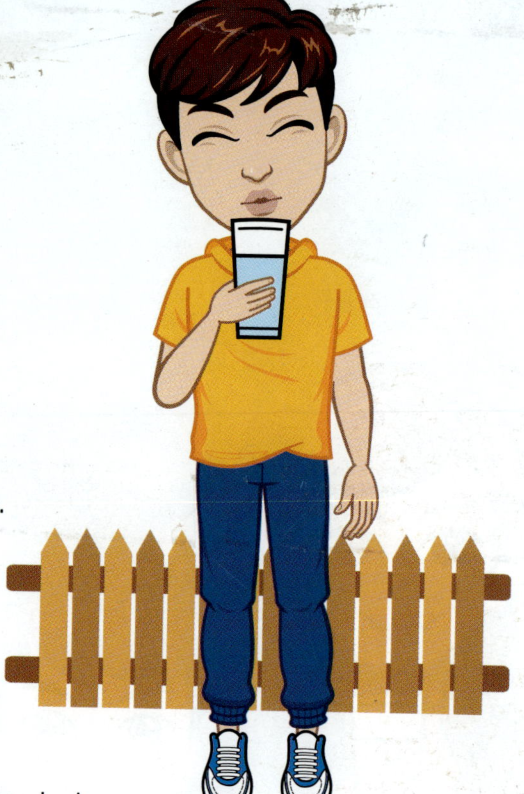

Suggestion Box

- Drink a lot of water.
- Take more liquids but not in the form of tea, coffee and cold drinks but in the forms of sherbet, coconut water, thin buttermilk and vegetable juices.
- Have more fruits which have more content of waters like oranges, muskmelons, cucumbers, and watermelons.
- Drink more water in summer than in winter.
- If you are perspiring due to physical exercise, then drink more water.

Dietary fiber

Kids, believe us, all our diseases originate from our unhealthy Gastro intestrial tract (Stomach) – digestive system. If your digestive system is strong, you are strong.

Dietary fiber is a component of dietary plant material that cannot be digested by enzymes. It is made up of cellulose, hemicellulose and pectin.

There are two types of Fiber

- Insoluble dietary fiber – It is found in foods such as whole grains, wheat bran and vegetables. It is also found in fenugreek seeds. It has proved to be effective in reducing blood glucose and cholesterol level.
- Soluble dietary fiber – It is found in nuts, seeds, beans and lentils. It is also found in psyllium, a common fiber supplement.

Functions of Fiber

- It contributes to the bulk in the diet thereby reducing energy intake and helps to reduce weight.
- Provides fecal bulk; so, it is good for constipation.
- Stimulating peristalsis – fiber is essential for the movement of the bowel as it stimulates and contracts the intestine.

This has always been a negligible part in diet, but it is the most important part!

Suggestion Box

- You should eat at least 3 to 5 vegetables and fruits for your fiber need.
- High dietary fibre intake interferes in the absorption of iron, calcium, zinc and vitamins.
- So keep distance between fiber and calcium and iron intake.
- If you are taking high fiber diet, then ensure plenty of water intake.
- Dietary fiber increases the bacterial flora, killing the bad bacteria and increasing good bacteria.

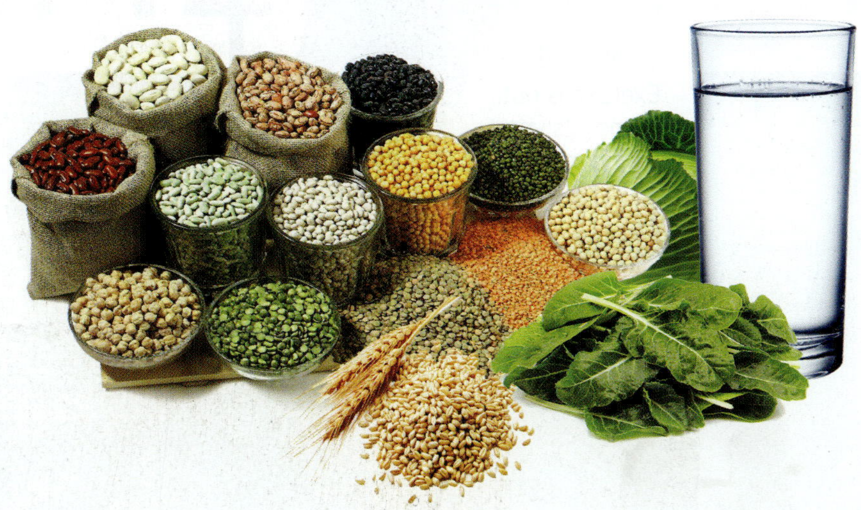

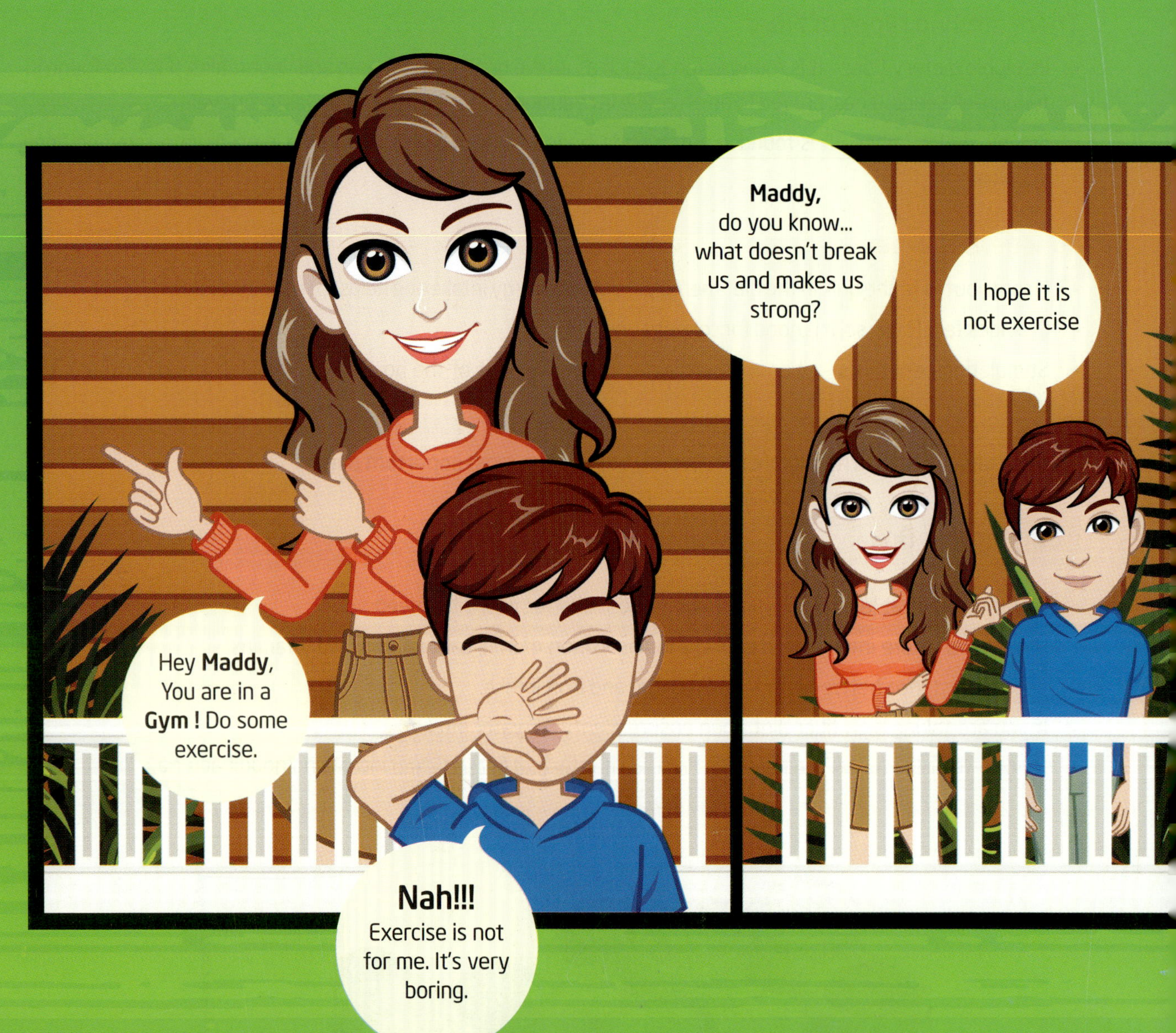

Maddy,
do you know...
what doesn't break
us and makes us
strong?

I hope it is
not exercise

Hey Maddy,
You are in a
Gym ! Do some
exercise.

Nah!!!
Exercise is not
for me. It's very
boring.

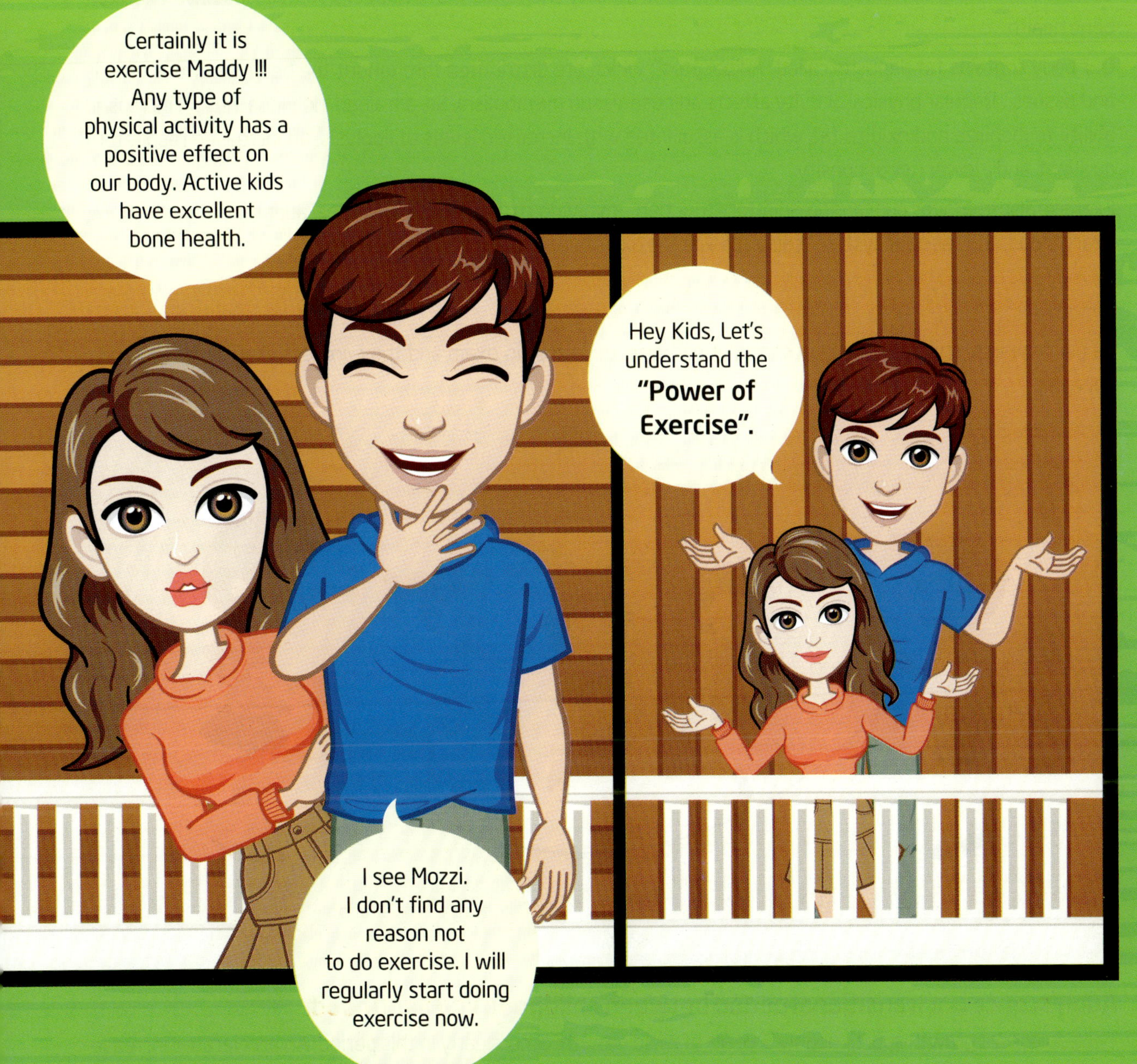

9. Power of Exercise

Lot of kids think "exercise" is boring.

But many studies have shown that, in children and adolescents, strength training can increase muscle strength, power, and endurance. Any type of physical activity has a positive effect on our body. In fact, active children and adolescents have greater bone mineral content and density than their inactive peers. Active kids have excellent bone health.

Our body contains fat deposits called "Adipocytes"; which are distributed throughout the body in various organs and tissues. Regular physical activity affects adipose tissue metabolism. So, a trained individual has an increased ability to mobilize and oxidize fat, which is associated with increased levels of lipolysis, an increased respiratory quotient, and a lower risk of obesity.

Exercise also improves our cardiorespiratory function - involving structural and functional adaptations in the lungs, heart, blood, and vascular system. It also impacts the oxidative capacity of skeletal muscles.

Fat Fact

As per research, children who play sports or exercise, do better in exam and they are less likely to have unruly behavior.

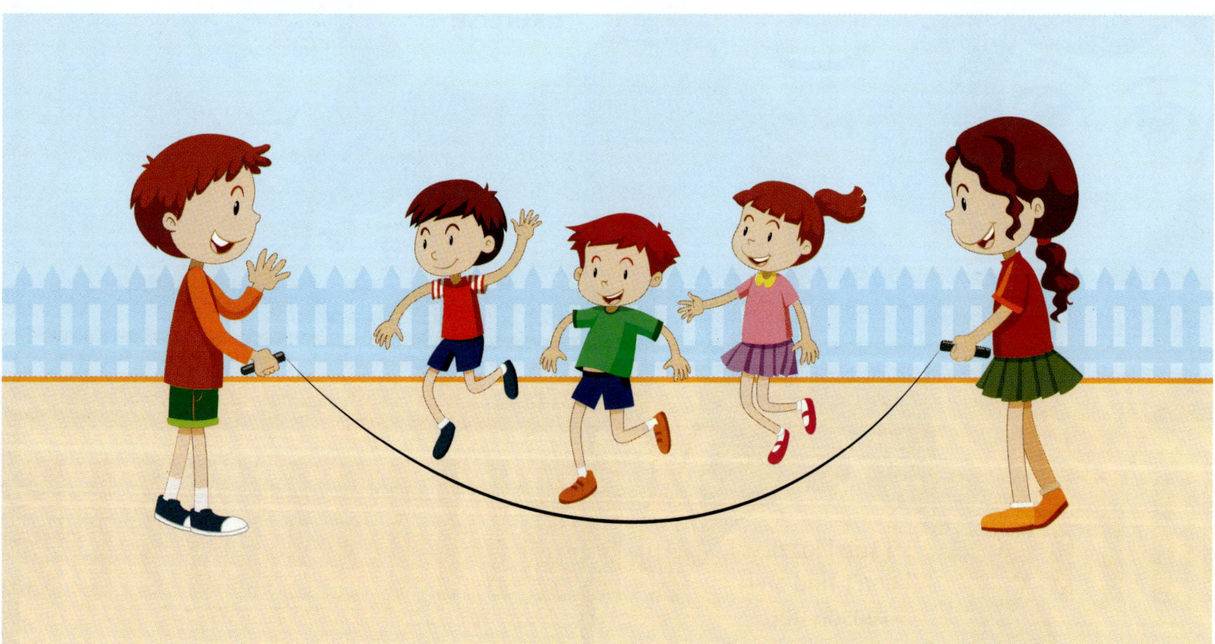

Adolescence is a transitional period between childhood and adulthood.

The adolescent growth spurt, roughly 3 years of rapid growth, occurs early in this period. An accelerated increase in stature is a hallmark, with about 20 percent of adult stature being attained during this period. Along with the rapid increase in height, other changes in body proportions occur that have important implications.

Suggestion Box

- If you really want good height, then do exercises such as jumping with high protein diet.
- You can do any physical exercise like dance and sports or strengthening exercise.
- Drink lots of water if you perspire a lot.

How to increase stamina in athletes / sports person/dancers by diet?

Nutrition for athletes / sports person / dancers is an evolved science and many factors are considered to achieve maximum results.

Eating for maximum performance includes eating food for the maintenance of optimum health, plus extra nutrients to achieve maximum performance.

Sports person feel that they can eat as much as they want to as they are very active and do exercise. But this is a wrong concept. Sports person need to pay more attention to nutrition.

Suggestion Box

- Meal timing and frequency is very important, so fix them according to your activity.
- Before going for exercise have some carbohydrates like peanut butter with bread / yoghurt plus oats/ banana/ dry fruits.
- During exercise have water sip by sip. Other options are coconut water with salt / lemon sharbat/ glucose water. After exercise remember there are 4 "R".
- R – RECOVERY- vitamins and minerals.
- R- REPAIR - protein.
- R – REHYDRATE – water.
- R – Replenish- complex carbohydrate.

So how to complete these FOUR "R's.

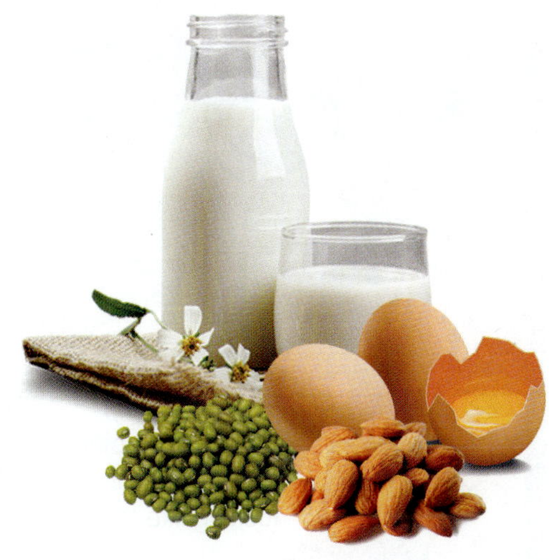

Options :

- One fruit with eggs or sprouts plus buttermilk.
- Rajgeera, lahi or Makhana
- Oat + milk+ fruit with some dry fruits.
- Sattu water with nut and seeds powder with fruits.
- Before competition you need carbohydrates to store glucose in your livers, but for this you need an expert's guidance.

Exercise Fact

Daily physical education in primary school appears to have a significant long term positive effect on exercise habit in women as compared to men. They are more active as they age.

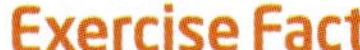

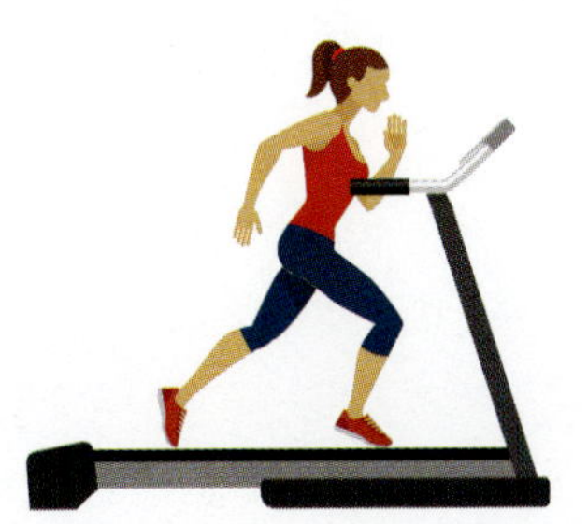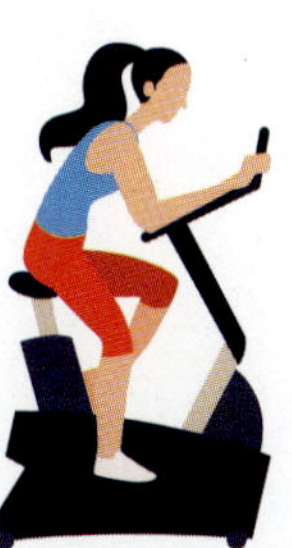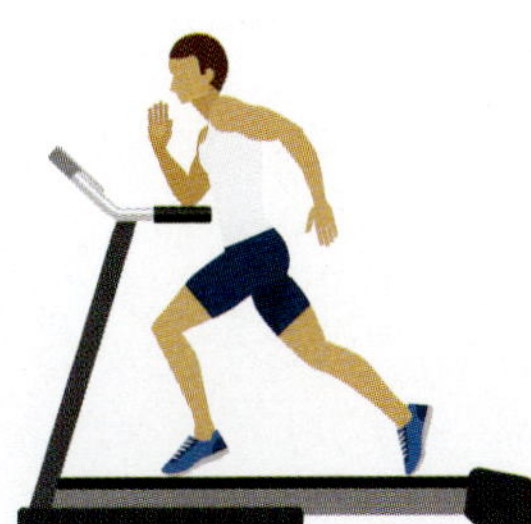

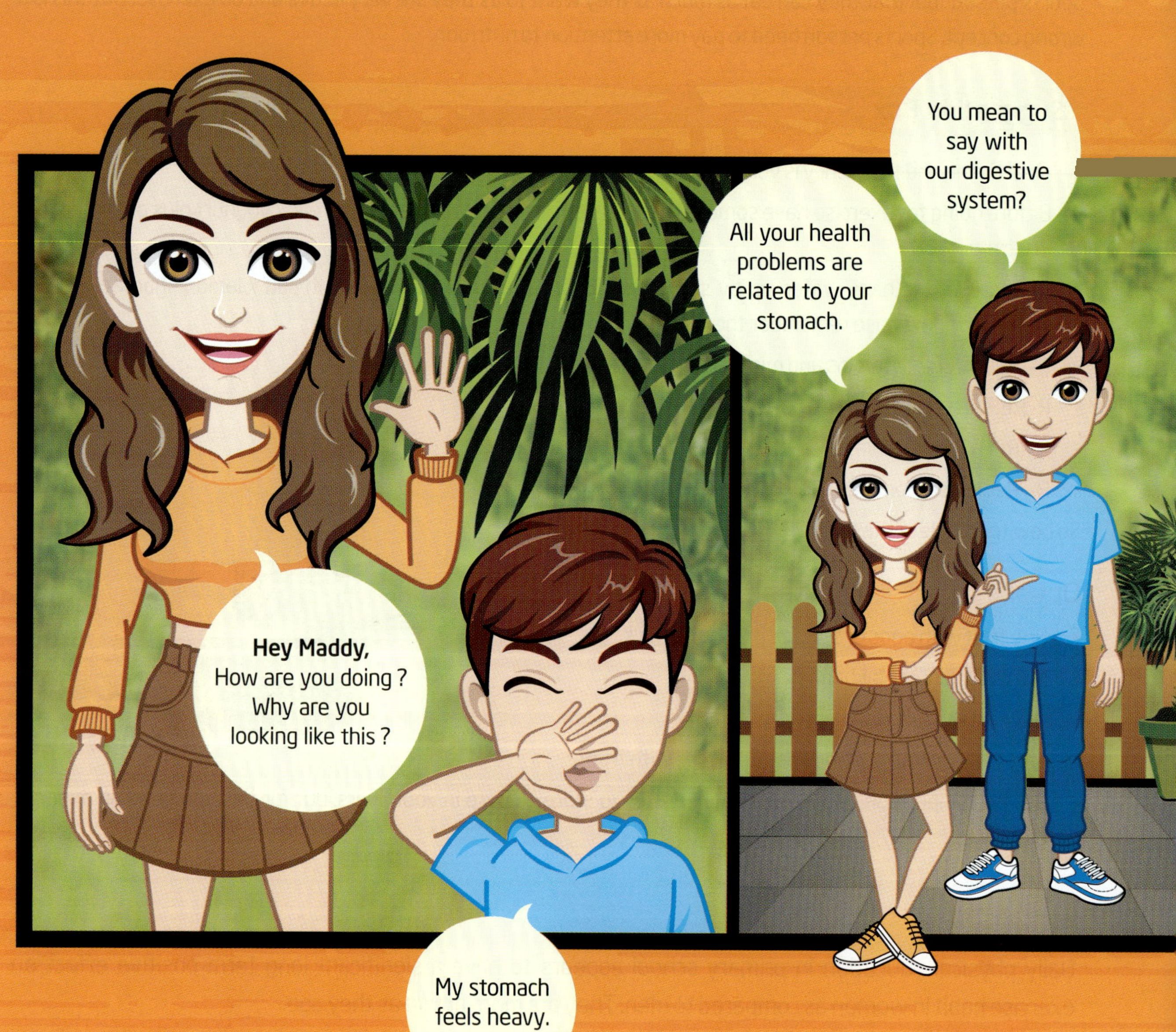

Hey Maddy, How are you doing ? Why are you looking like this ?
My stomach feels heavy.
All your health problems are related to your stomach.
You mean to say with our digestive system?

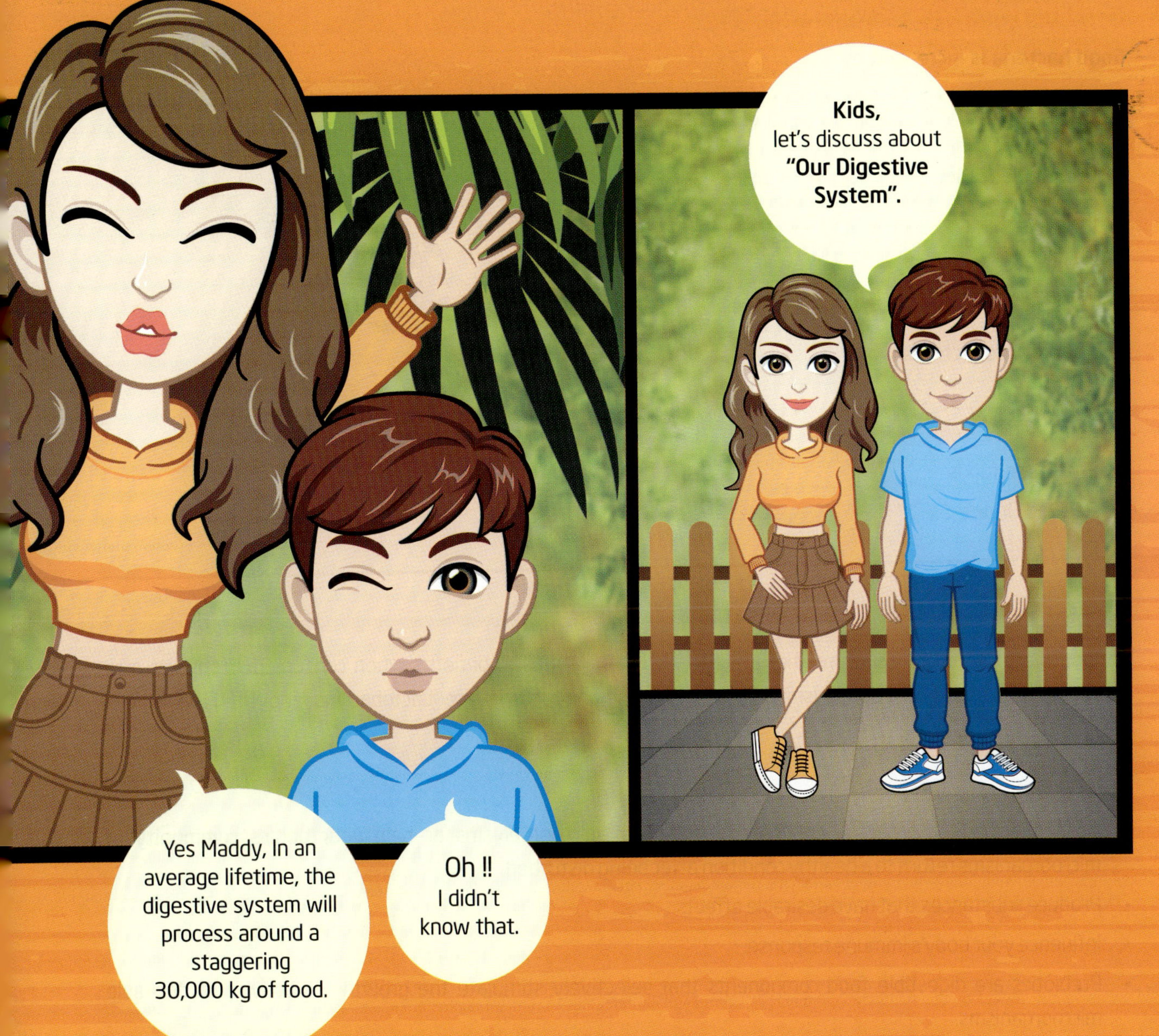

10. Our Digestive System

Digestive Fact

In an average lifetime, the digestive system will process a staggering 30,000 kg of Food.

Well, let us explain how it works. Our digestive system has good bacteria as well as bad bacteria. Up to 2kg of your body weight consists of bacteria. The average person is host to around four hundred different types of friendly bacteria, they mainly reside in the digestive tract. These good bacteria are the first line of defense against viruses and bacteria.

Good bacteria v/s bad bacteria

Good bacteria is increased by

- Water
- Vegetables
- Pre-probiotic Diets
- Fruits
- Balanced Diets
- Pickles

Bad bacteria is increased by

- Sugar
- Salt
- Processed foods
- Aerated Drinks
- Junk Food

Probiotics

Probiotics are live microorganisms that are intended to have health benefits when consumed. Probiotics may contain a variety of microorganisms. The most common bacteria are Lactobacillus and Bifid bacterium, Saccharomyces boulardii.

Functions

- Help your body maintain a healthy community of microorganisms or help your body's community of microorganisms return to a healthy condition after being disturbed.
- Produce substances that have desirable effects.
- Influence your body's immune response.
- Prebiotics are digestible food components that selectively stimulate the growth or activity of desirable microorganisms.
- Symbiotic are products that combine probiotics and prebiotics. It is available in the form of powder.

All these increase your digestibility which help in absorption of nutrients as well as immune system. Probiotics are in foods such as yogurt.

Prebiotics are in foods such as whole grains, bananas, greens, onions, garlic, soybeans.

Suggestion Box

- Yogurt has lot of lactobacillus which is good for body.

- Fresh curd (3-4 hrs.) gives you enough amount of good bacteria, named lactobacillus.

- Yogurt is good in lactose intolerance because of its digestibility.

- Homemade curd is made up of only lactobacillus bulgaricus and yogurt is made up of two or more different microorganisms.

- Eat fresh green leafy vegetables, bananas, and fresh pickles for healthy gut flora.

Dustbin

Remember our digestive system is not a dustbin, it's a temple. Our happiness and our diseases have a close relationship with our digestive system. So you have to decide what you want to put in it.

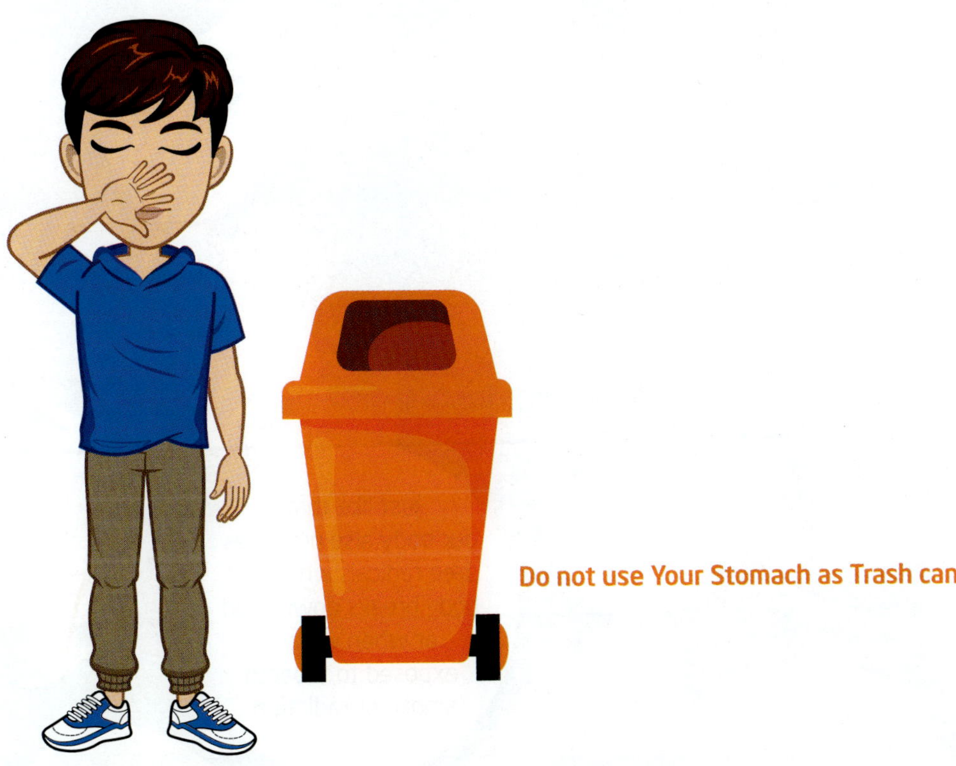

Suggestion Box

1. Eat slowly

2. Eat frequently

3. Chew properly

4. Eat fresh food

5. Eat local and seasonal fruits and vegetables

6. Eat 2 hrs. before bedtime

7. Limit your fast food and junk food as it weakens your digestive system

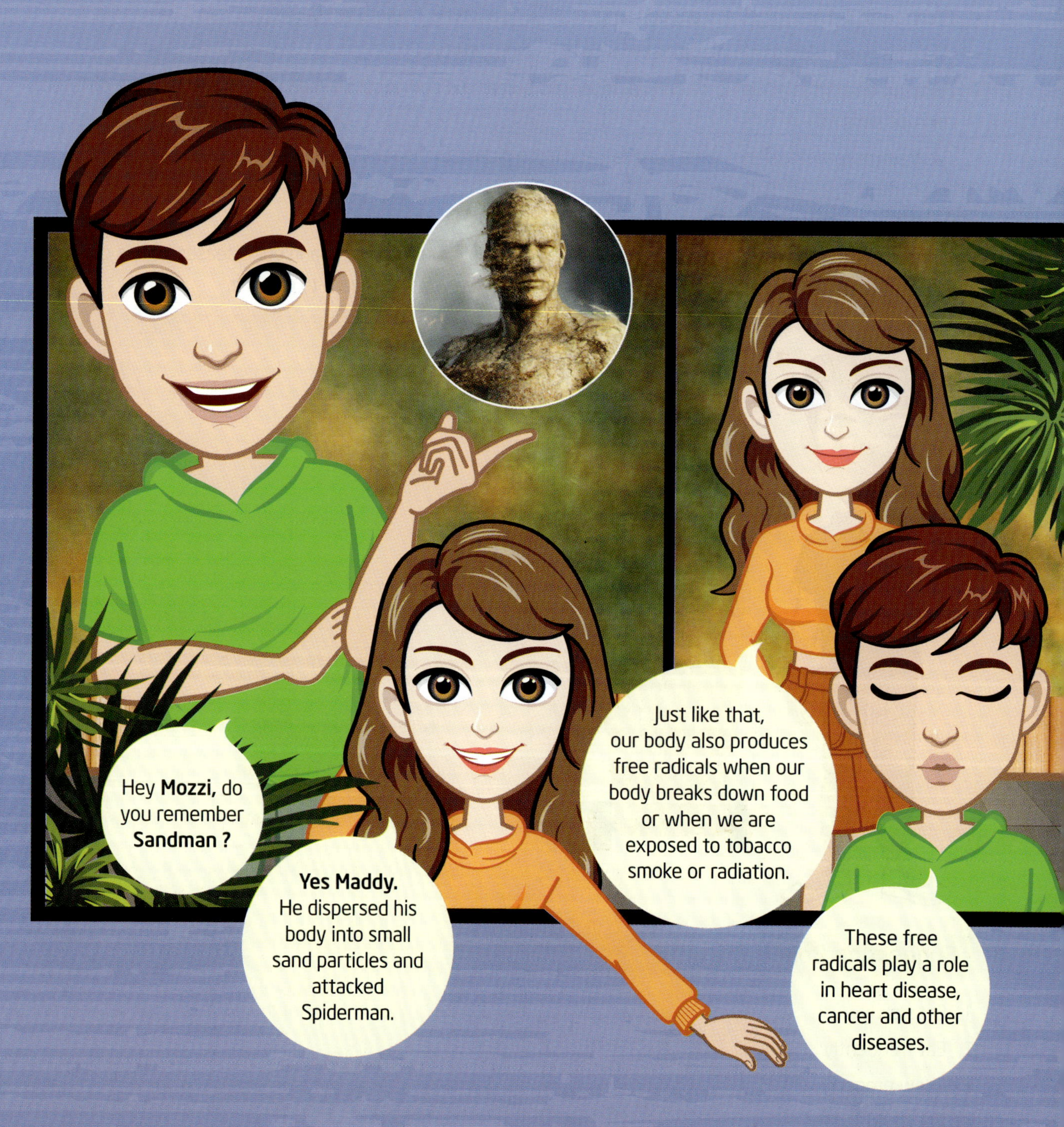

Hey Mozzi, do you remember Sandman ?
Yes Maddy. He dispersed his body into small sand particles and attacked Spiderman.
Just like that, our body also produces free radicals when our body breaks down food or when we are exposed to tobacco smoke or radiation.
These free radicals play a role in heart disease, cancer and other diseases.

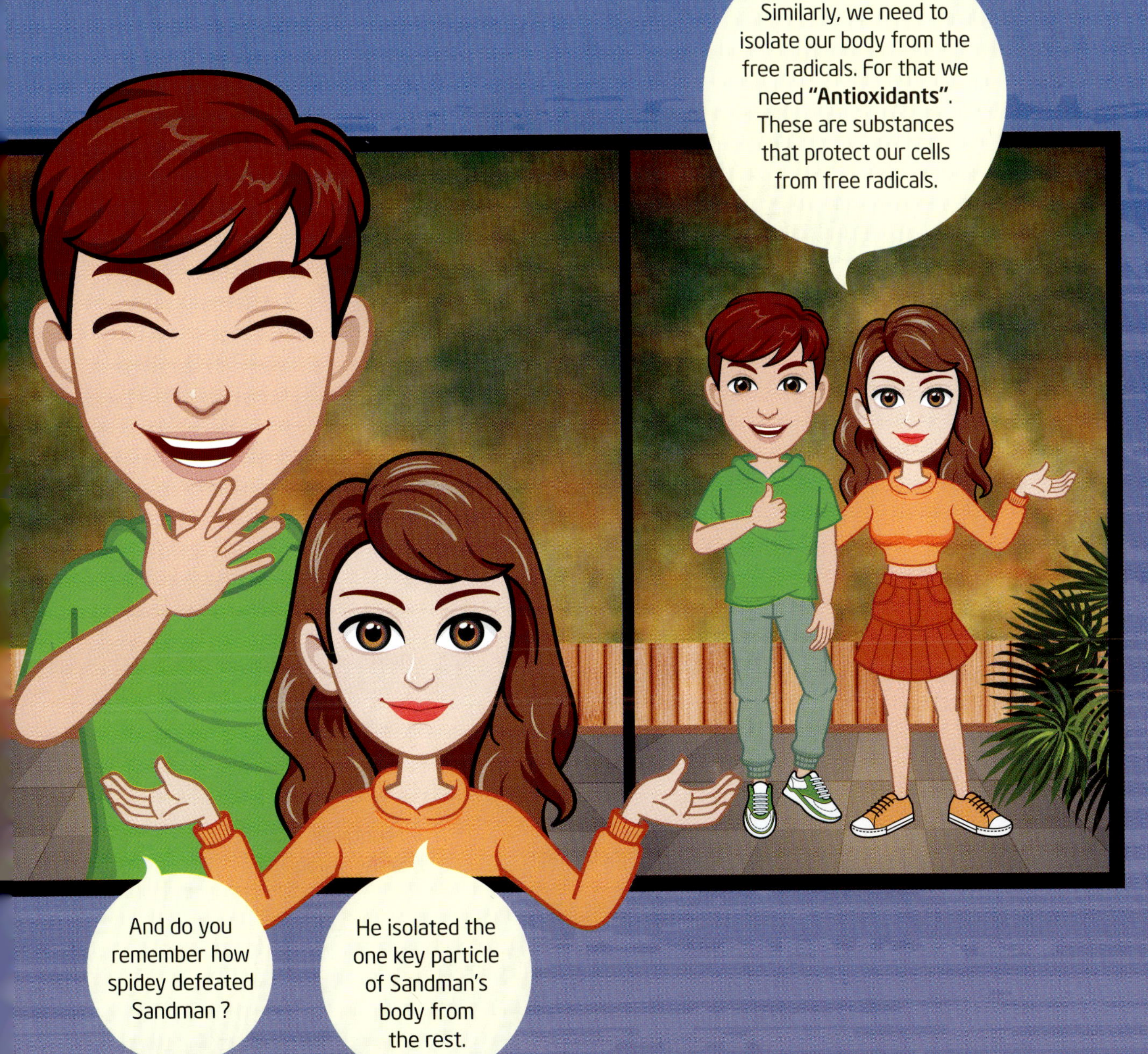

11. Antioxidants

Antioxidants, such as vitamins C and E and Vitamin A (carotenoids) may help protect cells from damage caused by free radicals. Other naturally occurring antioxidants include flavonoids, tannins, phenols and lignans.

Plant-based foods are the best sources. These include fruits, vegetables, whole grains, nuts, seeds, herbs and spices, and even cocoa.

As a bonus, fruits, vegetables and whole grains high in antioxidants are also typically high in fiber, low in saturated fat and cholesterol, and good sources of vitamins and minerals.

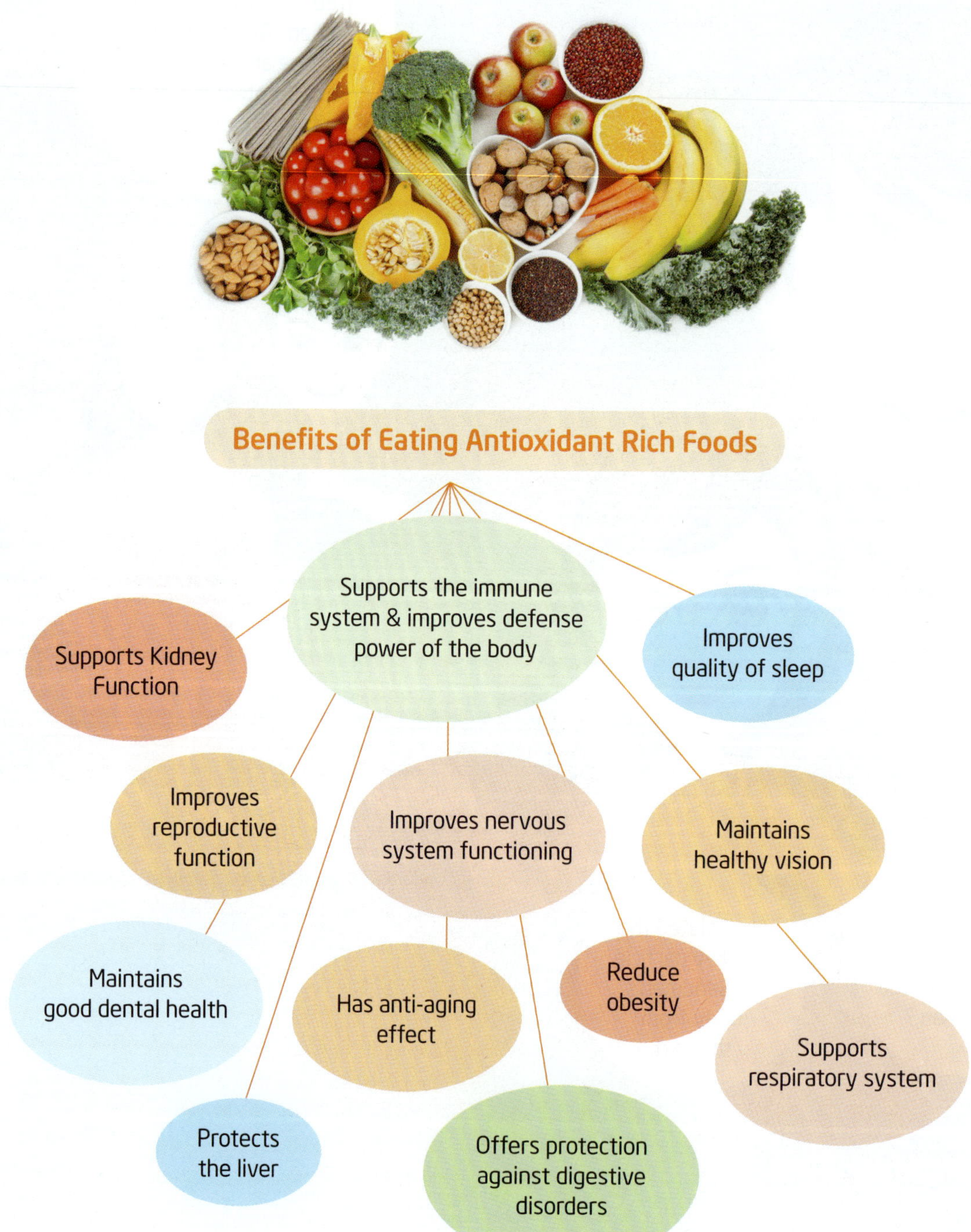

Indian Foods rich in antioxidants

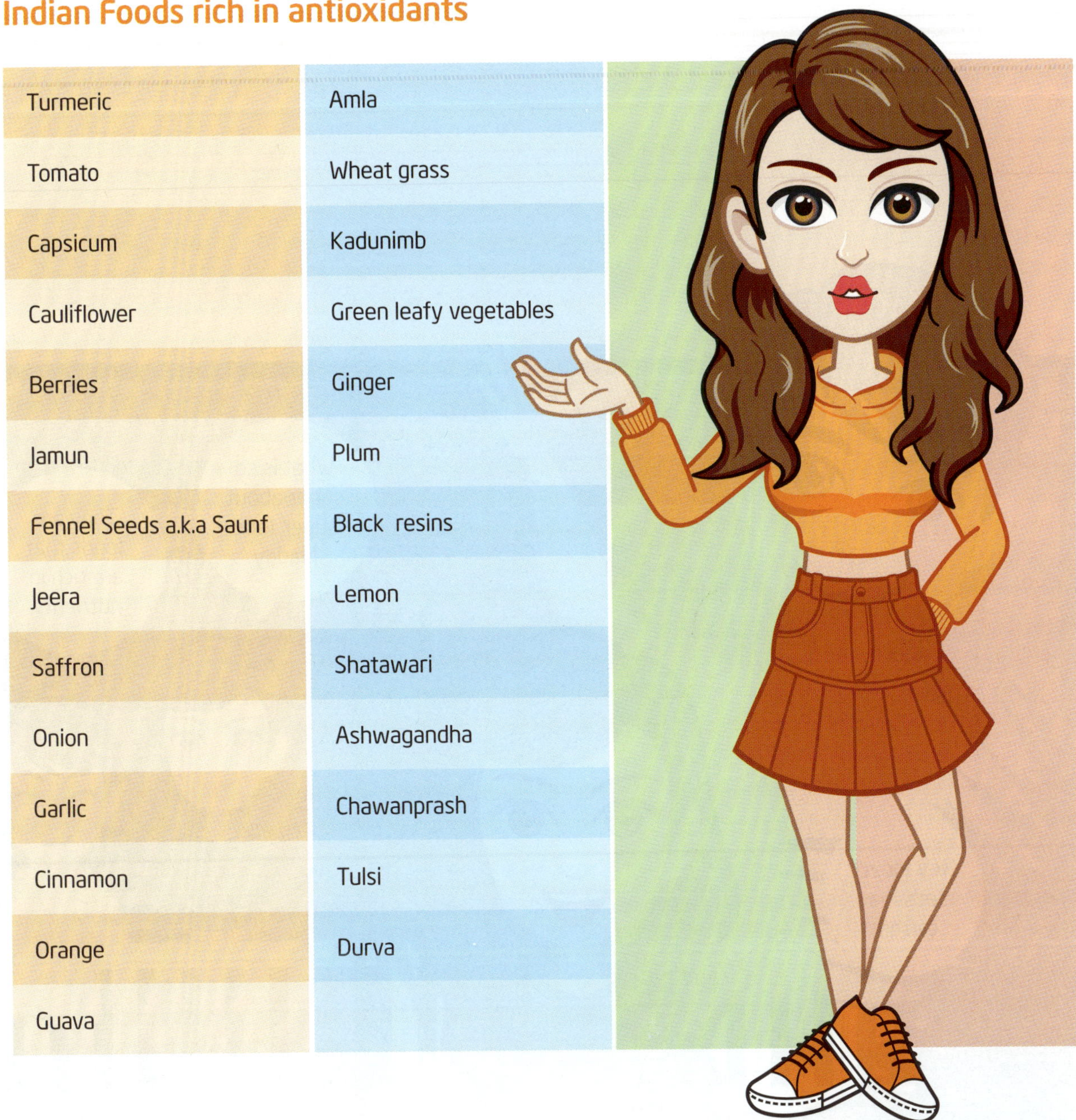

Turmeric	Amla
Tomato	Wheat grass
Capsicum	Kadunimb
Cauliflower	Green leafy vegetables
Berries	Ginger
Jamun	Plum
Fennel Seeds a.k.a Saunf	Black resins
Jeera	Lemon
Saffron	Shatawari
Onion	Ashwagandha
Garlic	Chawanprash
Cinnamon	Tulsi
Orange	Durva
Guava	

Suggestion Box

- Eat dark colour vegetables-darker=more antioxidants.
- Try different dark coloured fruits and vegetables every day to get maximum antioxidants.
- Use more spices in your diet like cloves, turmeric, black pepper and cinnamon. Add it to your salad, milk, or beverages.
- Try having more raw vegetables and fruits.

Omega 3 fatty acids are a good source of antioxidants.

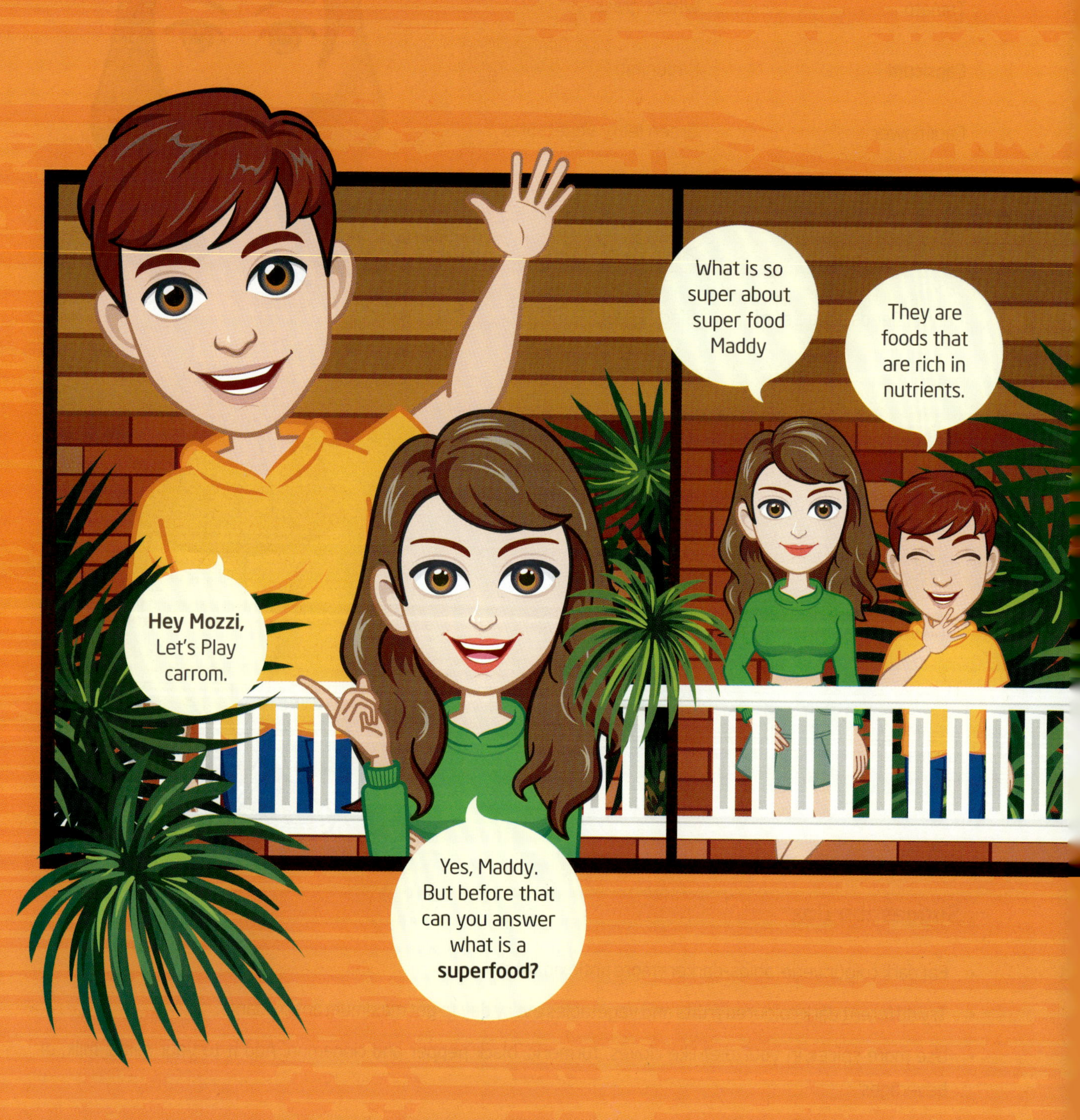
Hey Mozzi, Let's Play carrom.
Yes, Maddy. But before that can you answer what is a superfood?
What is so super about super food Maddy
They are foods that are rich in nutrients.

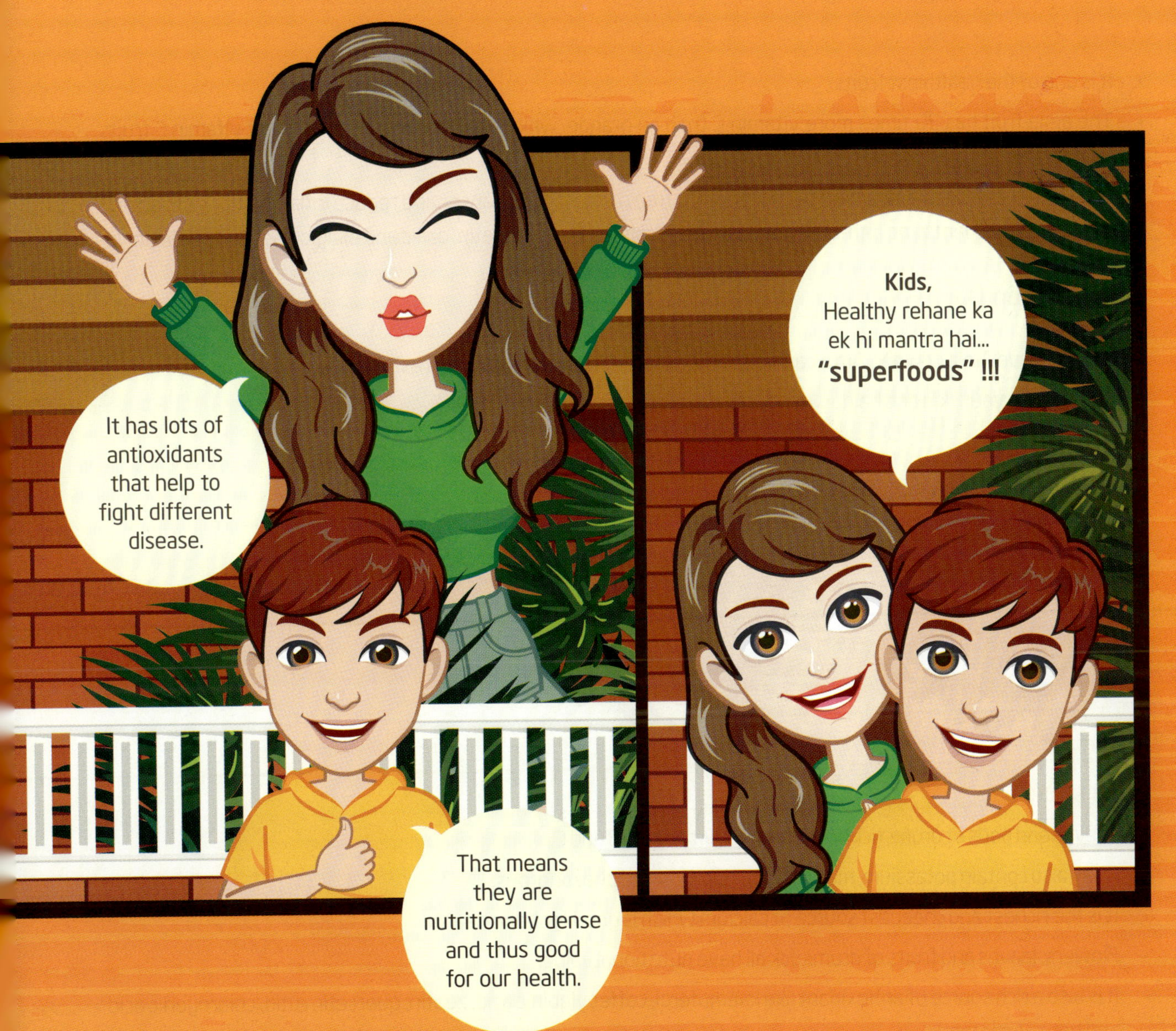

12. "Super" Foods

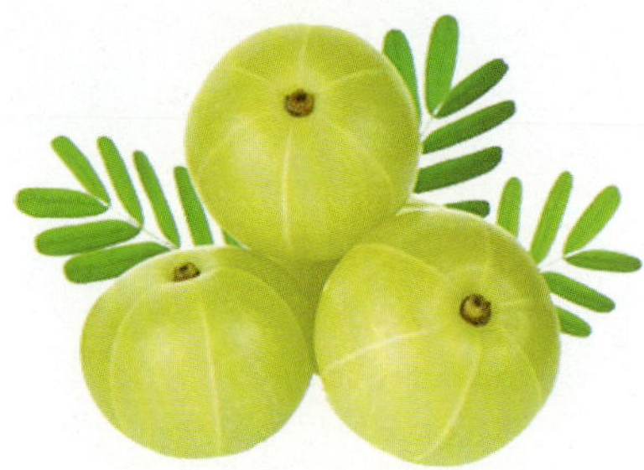

Amla

- It is one of the healthiest fruits.
- The amla fruit has 30 times more vitamin C than an orange, which makes it one of the richest vitamin C fruits available.
- Research has proven that amla can help prevent free radicals, fight cancer and reduce inflammations because it is rich in antioxidants and anti-inflammatory chemicals such as quercetin, gallic and ellagic acids and corilagin.

Suggestion Box

- You can have Amla powder, Amla candies, Amla juice, but the best option is fresh Amla.
- It's good for your skin and hair.

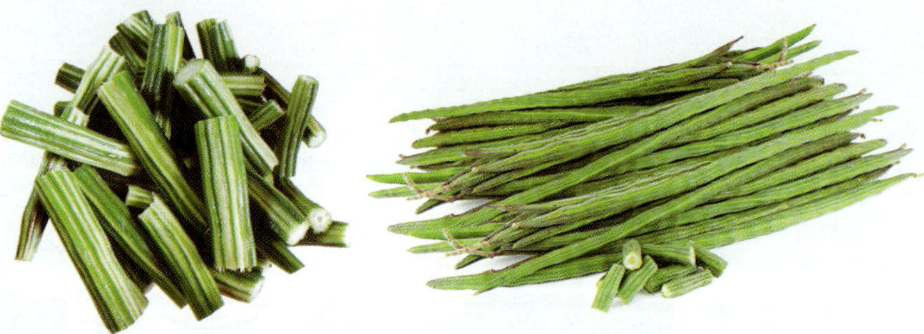

Drumstick

- Leaves and pods of drumstick are sources of vitamin A, B and C.
- They also contain potassium, magnesium, zinc, iron and phosphorous.
- It is the richest and cheapest source of calcium which is good for bone health.
- Flowers, leaves and fruits of drumstick all have nutritional value.
- It is also a rich source of antioxidant like kaempferol, caffeoylquinic acid, zeatin, quercetin rutin, chlorogenic acid and beta – sitosterol.

Suggestion Box

- Moringa is available in the form of powder, it can be used in water, mixed in parathas or pakoras.
- You can eat drumstick leaves in the form of vegetable or parathas because it's a good source of calcium. You should have it for your healthy bones.

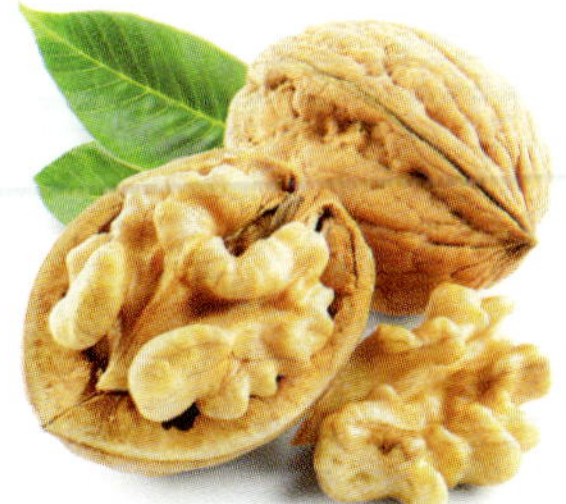

Walnuts

- Walnuts are made up of 65% fat and about 15% of protein. They're low in carbs and rich in fiber.
- It also has copper, folic acid, phosphorus, vitamin B6, manganese, and vitamin E.
- It's a powerhouse of antioxidants.
- It contains ellagic acid, catechin, melatonin, and phytic acid.
- Walnuts contain omega 3 fatty acids which help to prevent heart diseases as well as improve brain functions.
- It reduces the risk of cancer.

Suggestion Box

- Have walnuts early in the morning as they are easy to digest (Avoid if you are allergic).
- Having 5-6 walnuts every day is good for your memory. They increase your learning skills which help in your studies.

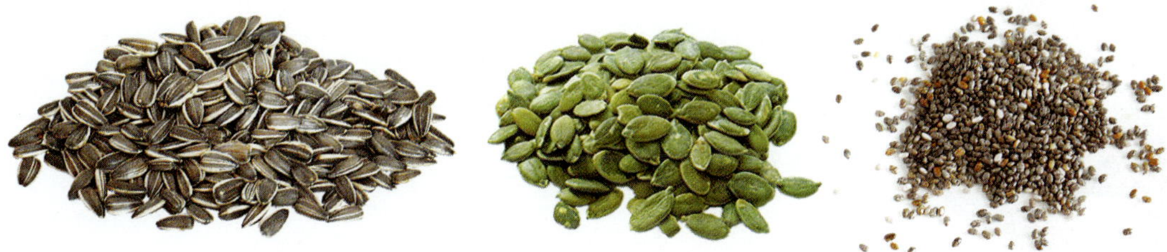

Seeds

- Seeds include sesame, poppy, sunflower, pumpkin, chia, flax seeds.
- They contain mixtures of proteins, fiber and fats, including mono unsaturated fatty acids, polyunsaturated fatty acids, and omega-3 fatty acids.
- They also contain zinc, magnesium, iron, calcium, copper, selenium, phosphorus and potassium.
- They are rich in some Vitamins like B1, B2, B3 and Vitamin E.
- They are rich in phytochemicals which act as antioxidants.
- Some seeds contain lignans which help to reduce cholesterol and risk of cancer.

Suggestion Box

- You can add poppy seeds and sesame seeds in your salads or vegetables.
- Chia seeds or sabja can be soaked in water before consuming.
- Flax seeds – add in your roti and salad.

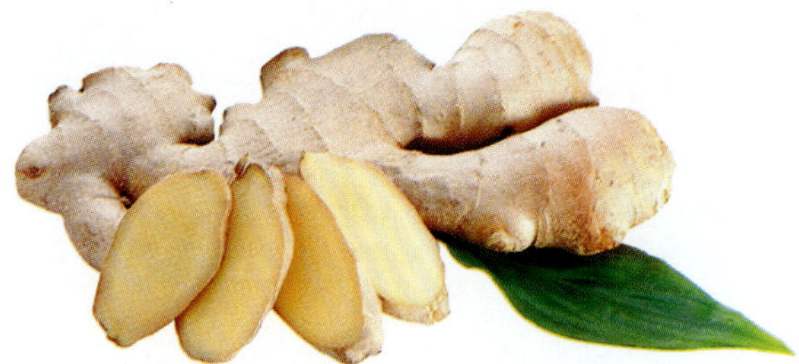

Ginger

- Ginger has gingerol bioactive compound which is anti-inflammatory as well as antioxidant. It decreases nausea.
- It reduces muscle pain and soreness.
- It has enzymes which help to reduce indigestion problem.
- It is good for heart diseases. It reduces cholesterol specially LDL
- It gives relives from cough and cold.
- It has anticancer properties as it contains gingerol.

Suggestion Box

- Take two teaspoon ginger & tulsi juice, add 1 tea spoon honey. It helps to boost your immunity.

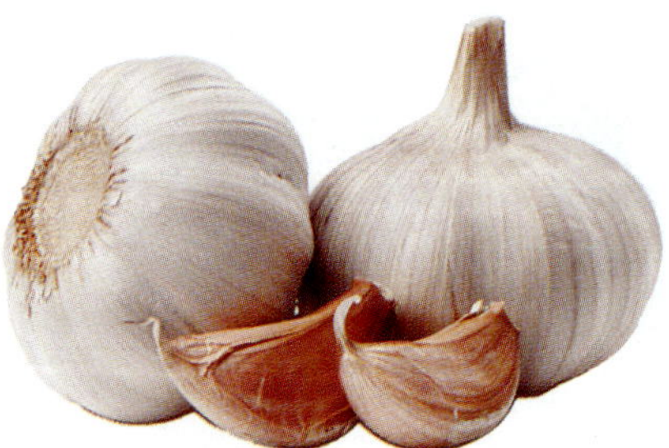

Garlic

- It has high % of minerals and vitamins and also contains traces of chlorine, iodine, phosphorus and Sulphur.
- In Russia, it is considered to be more powerful than penicillin.
- Garlic produces a chemical called allicin which has antimicrobial, antibiotic, antiviral properties, but it is released when we crush the garlic and that's why we should always use crushed garlic.
- Garlic improves HDL, lowers cholesterol, prevents blood clotting.
- It has antiseptic, antifungal, antibiotic effects which boosts your immune system.

Suggestion Box

- Eat at least 3 raw cloves in crushed form everyday (releases allicin).
- You can add it in your salad.
- You can add in your chutney.

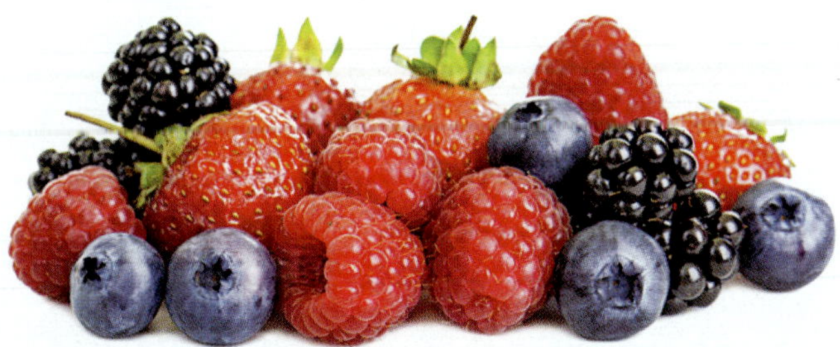

Berries

- Berries include strawberries, blueberries, blackberries, cranberries, Indian berries.
- Berries are good source of different antioxidants like anthocyanins, ellagic acids, and resveratrol, which help keep free radicals under control.
- It is high in soluble fiber which helps to reduce the weight and helps in constipation.
- It is a rich source of vitamin C.
- It contains ellagic acid which helps to reduce the wrinkles.
- Because of anthocyanins it helps protect against cancer

Suggestion Box

- They are seasonal fruits so eat only when they are available.
- They are full of antioxidants.
- Every day you should have at least 10-20 berries.

In India we get Indian berries in winter season.

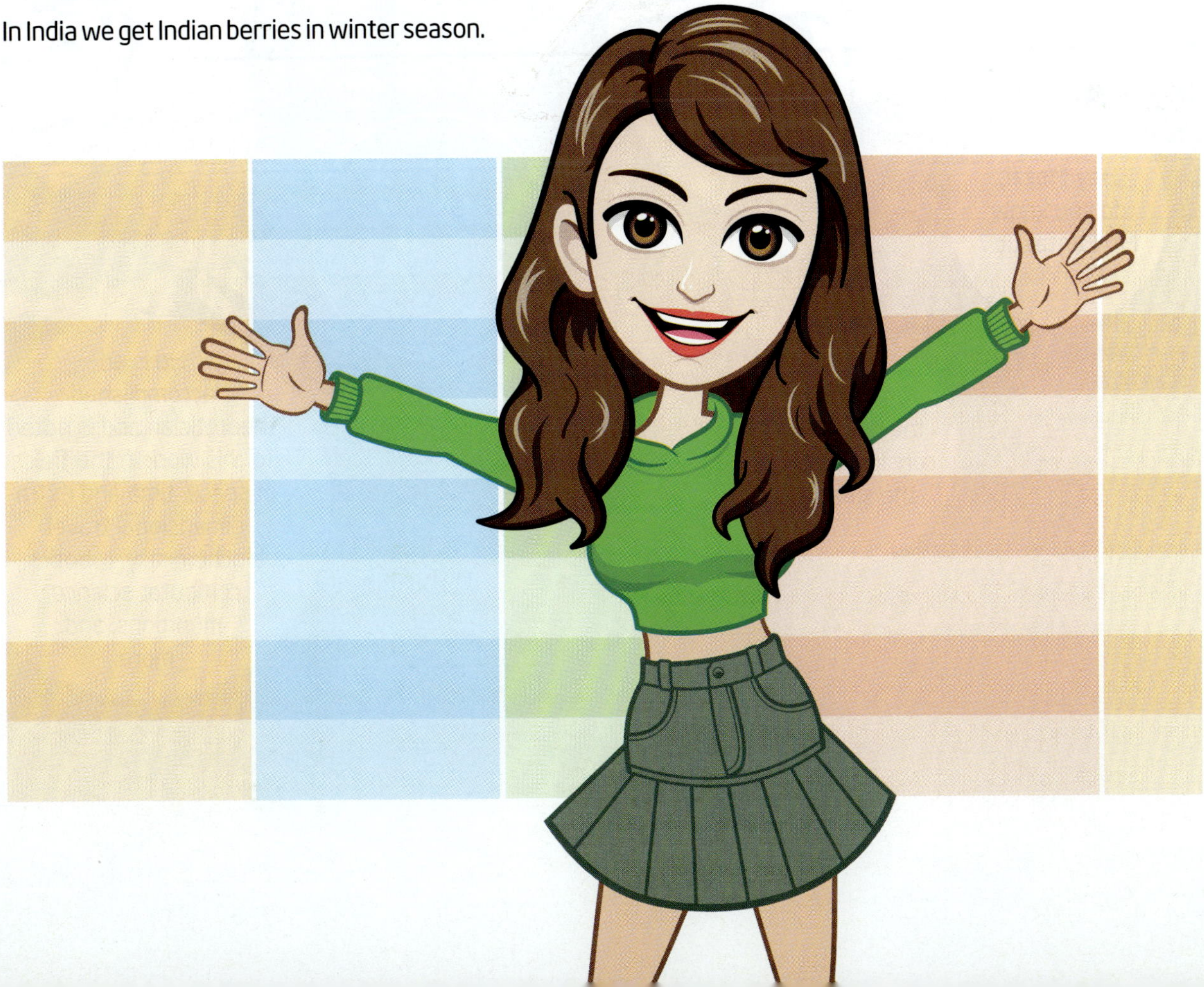

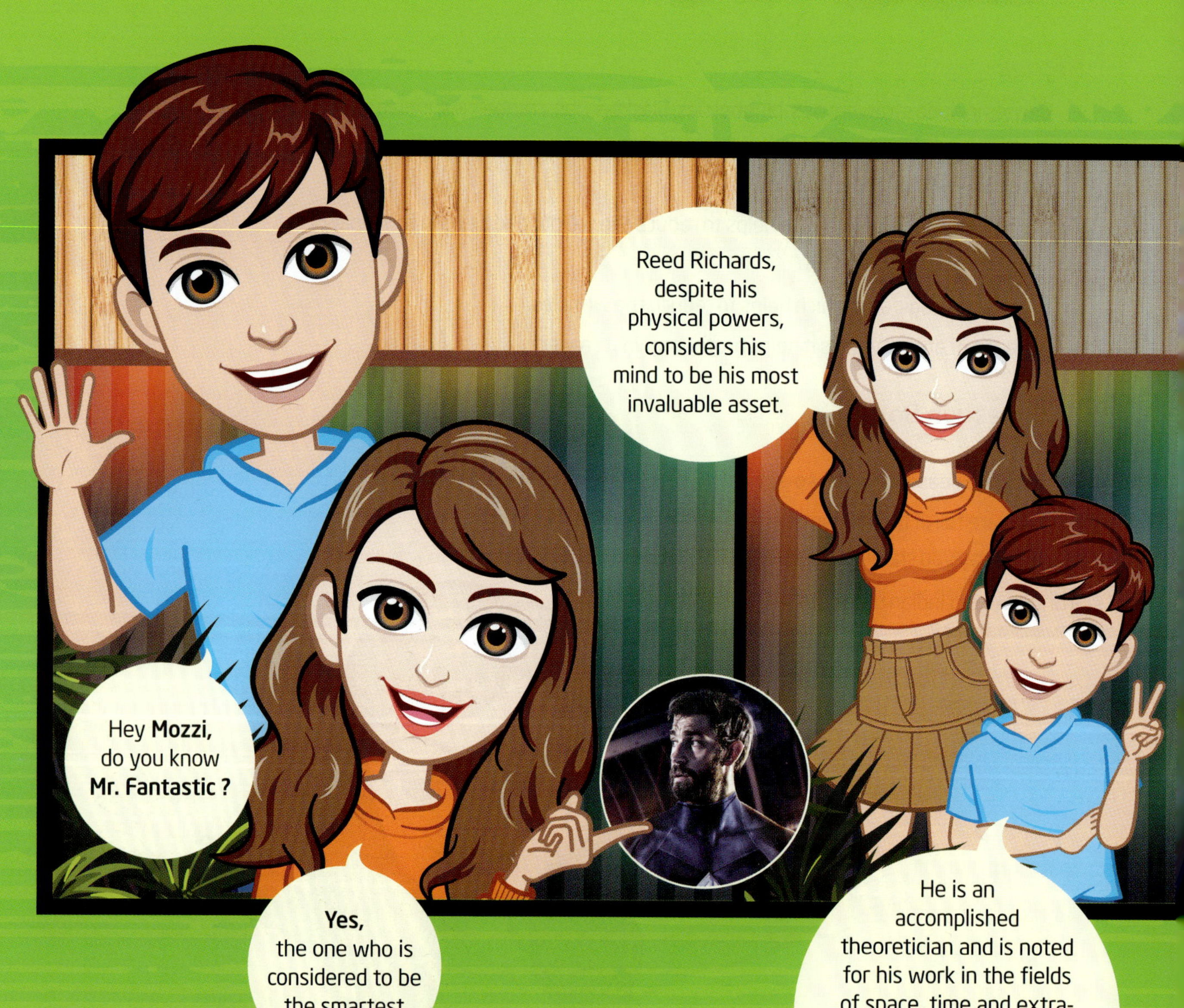

Hey Mozzi, do you know Mr. Fantastic ?
Reed Richards, despite his physical powers, considers his mind to be his most invaluable asset.
Yes, the one who is considered to be the smartest
He is an accomplished theoretician and is noted for his work in the fields of space, time and extra-dimensional travel, biochemistry, robotics, computer science, munitions, and more.

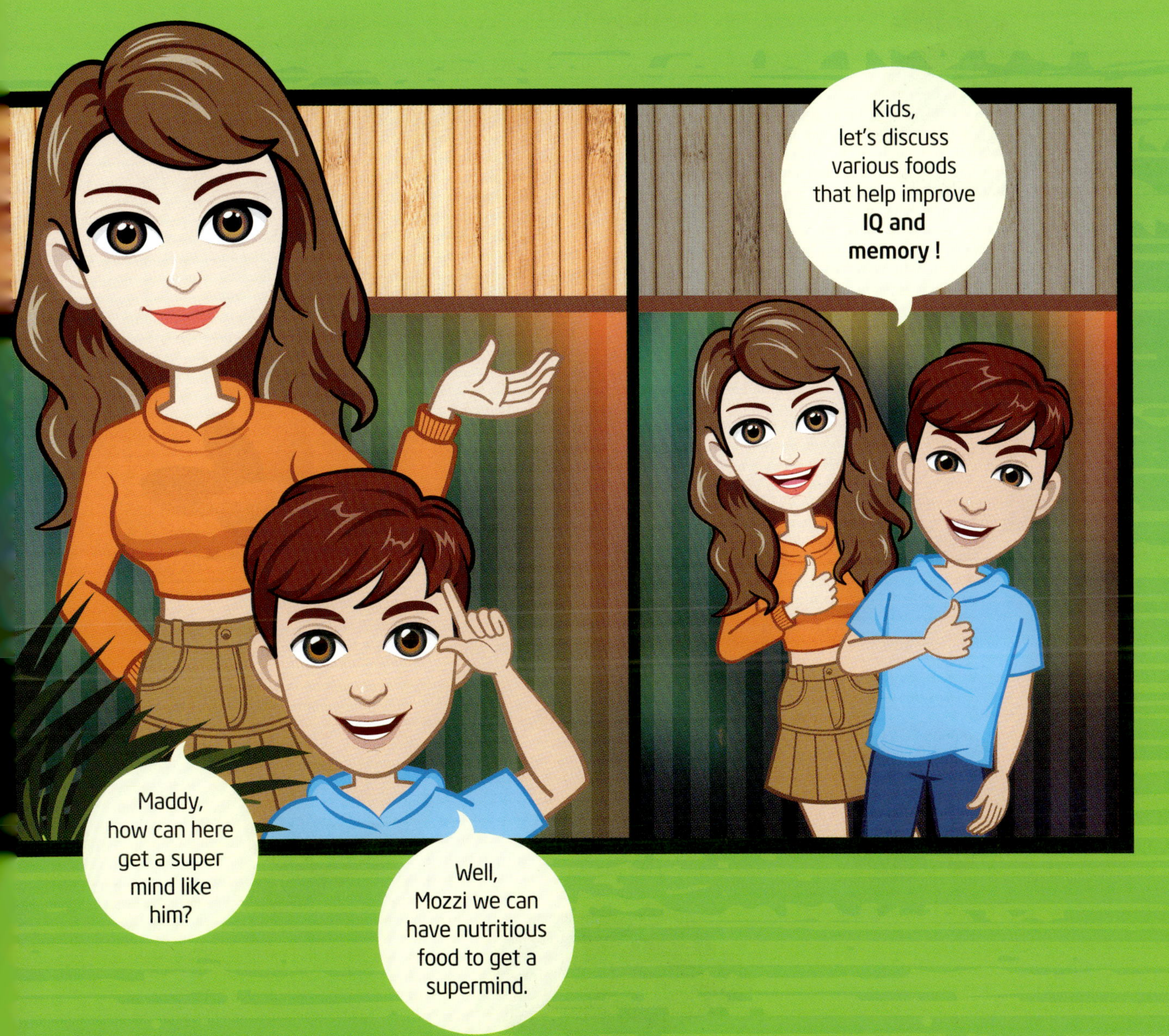

13. How to improve our IQ / Memory ?

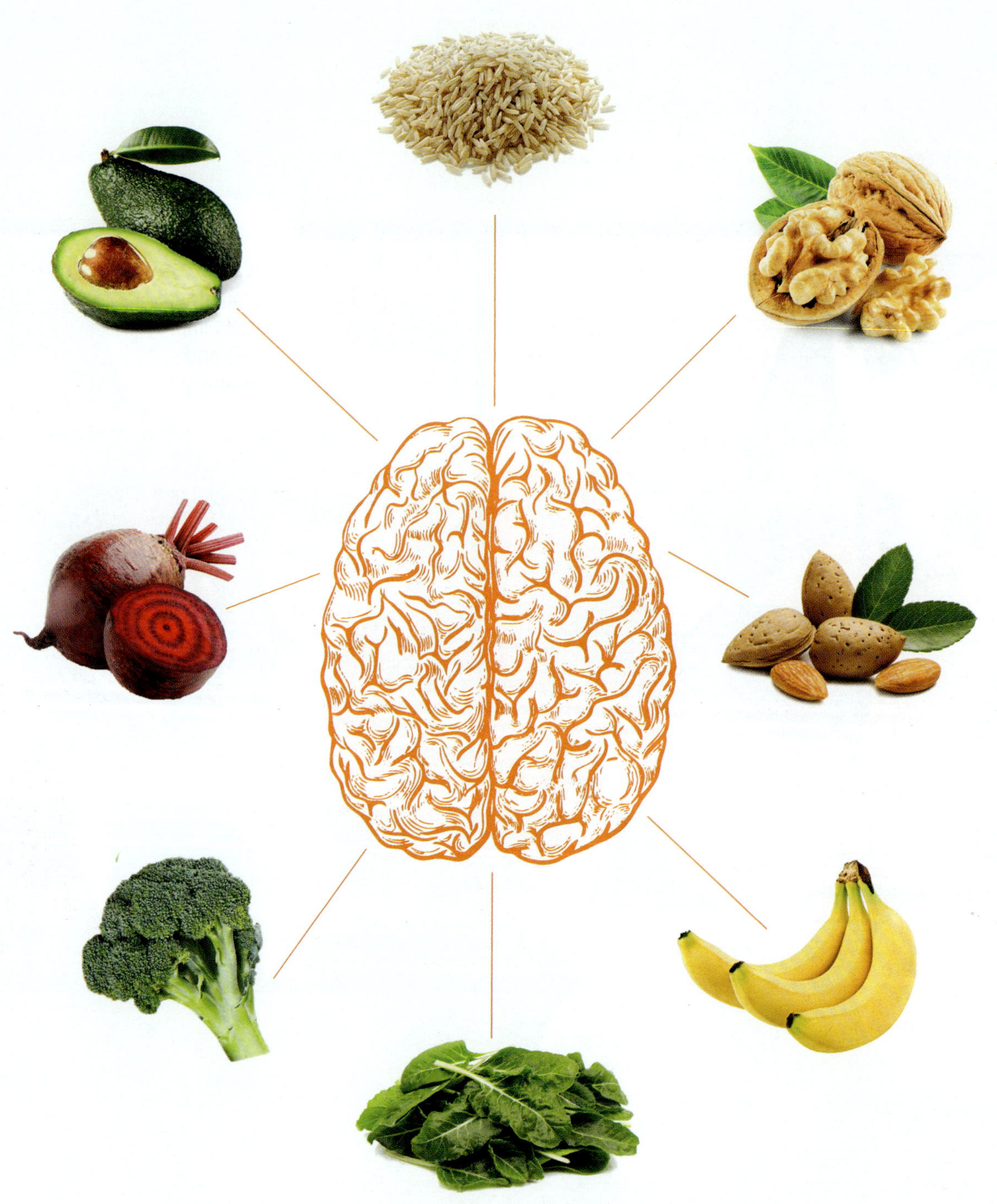

We can have all the food items listed below, to improve our IQ and memory !

- Grape fruit – It has flavonoid and polyphenol compound which improves memory; especially verbal learning.
- Nuts and seeds - They have a good amount of omega 3 and 6 fatty acids which are good for brain. Funny part is walnuts actually looks like a brain and are really good for the brain too
- Berries - All kind of berries help to improve memory.
- Fish – It is the richest source of omega 3 fatty acid which helps to increase IQ level.
- Cabbage, cauliflower, broccoli – They slow down brain aging.
- Nitric oxide - It improves brain blood flow. Beet juice (2 cups) and spinach are a good source of nitric oxide which is good for brain.
- Aerobic Exercise have recently been shown to have positive effects on the structure and functions of the brain.
- Beet juice and exercise develop brain network.
- Avocado, eggs, dark green leafy vegetables and spinach – They are good sources of 'Leutine'. It is present in the eyes and brain which help to reduce brain aging. Leutine can be modified by dietary intake which helps to improve writing and math.
- Finally, spinach is great for our brain!

Brain Food

Snacks That'll Boost Your Energy and Focus / As excerpted from fast company

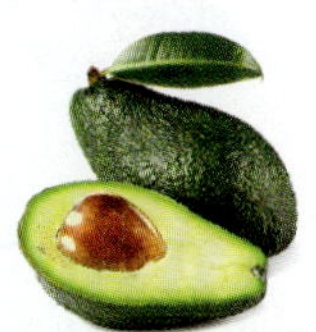

Avocado

As if we needed another reason to smear it on our toast every morning, it help with cognition.

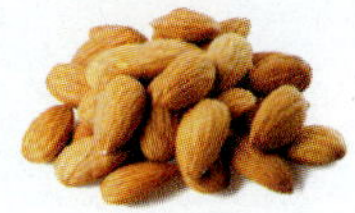

Almonds

The healthy fats in nuts help your brain process information and make connections.

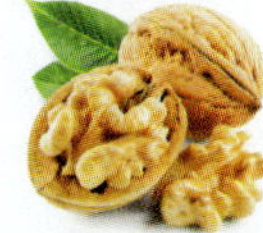

Walnuts

For better mental speed and accuracy.

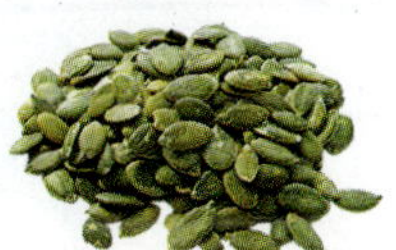

Pumpkin Seeds

Throw them into trail mix with some almonds and dark chocolate for a brain-boosting snack.

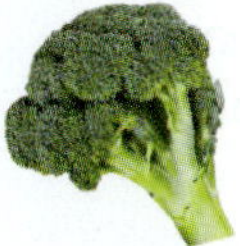

Broccoli

Mix in into a stir-fry bring it for lunch and improve your cognitive function.

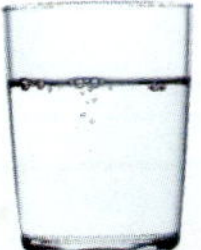

Water

Water improves every single bodily function, including quick thinking and focus.

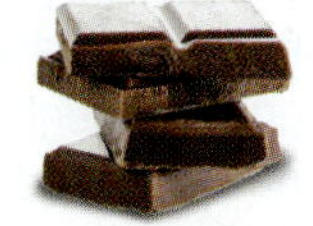

Dark Chocolate

It improves focus and energy, fights stress and is delicious.

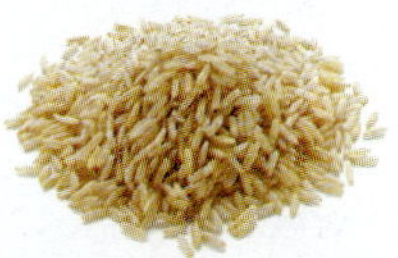

Brown Rice

Cross two off the list-avocado sushi with brown rice. Done.

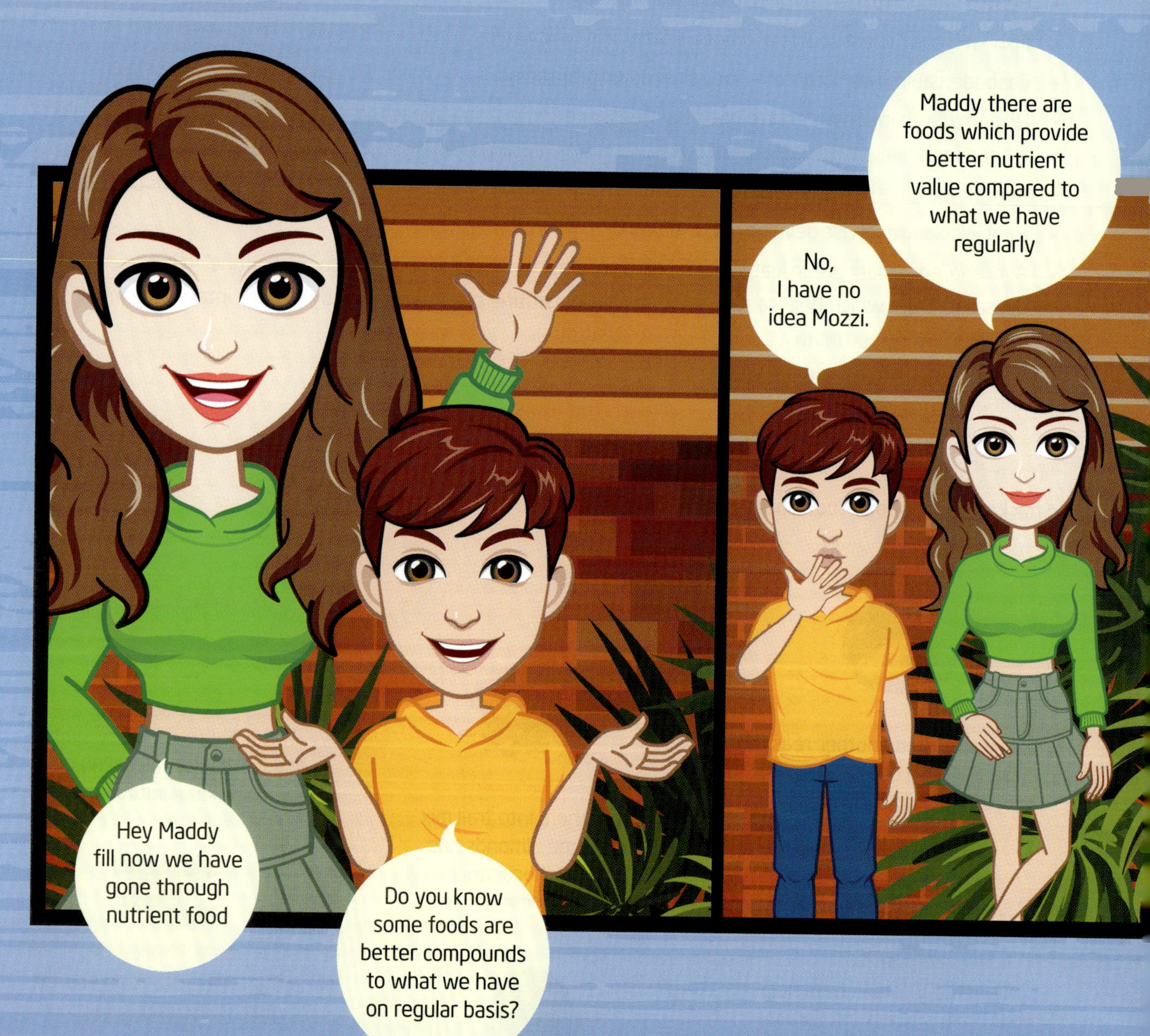

Maddy there are foods which provide better nutrient value compared to what we have regularly
No, I have no idea Mozzi.
Hey Maddy fill now we have gone through nutrient food
Do you know some foods are better compounds to what we have on regular basis?

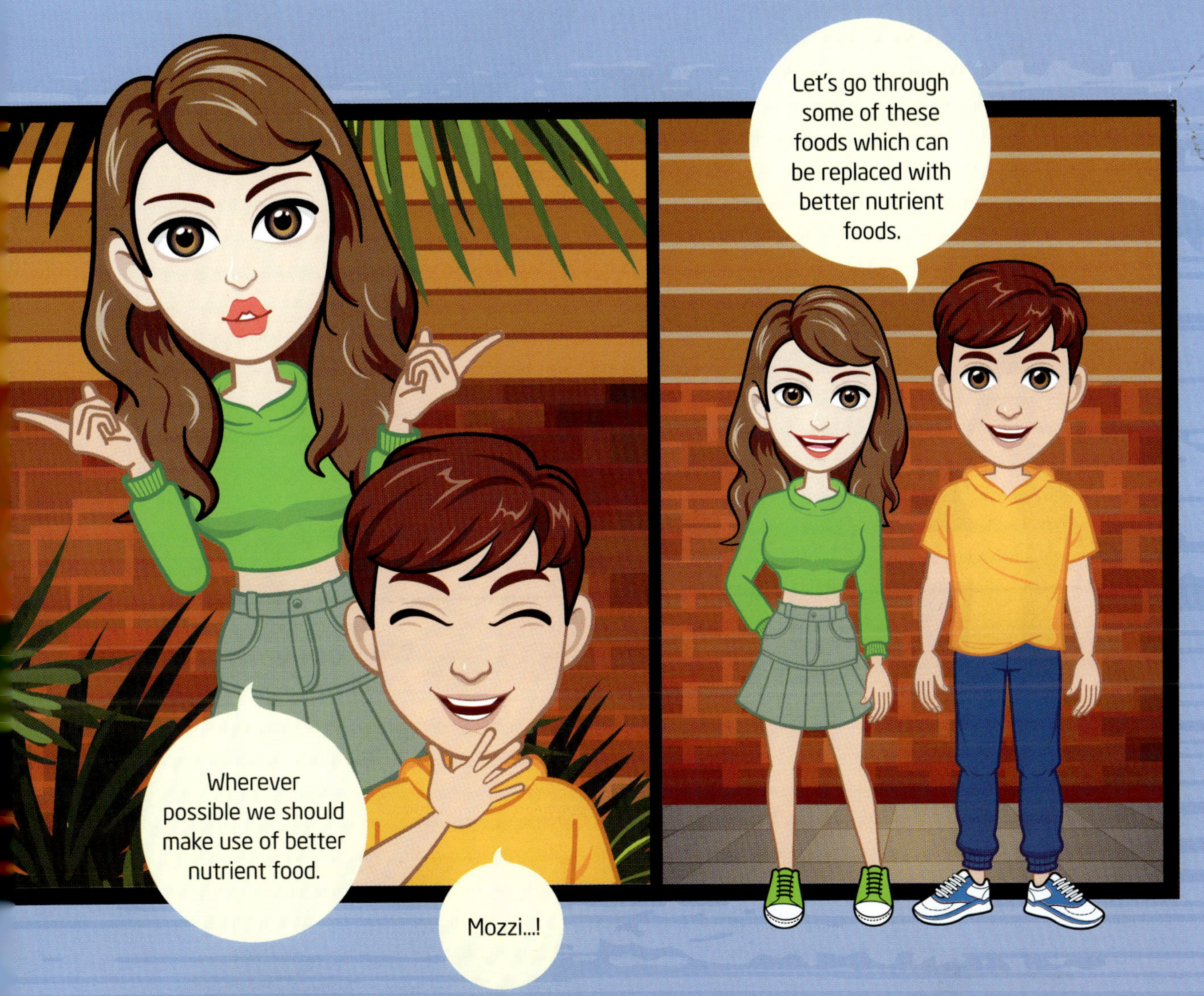

14. Swapping the Foods

White Sugar to Jaggery and Honey

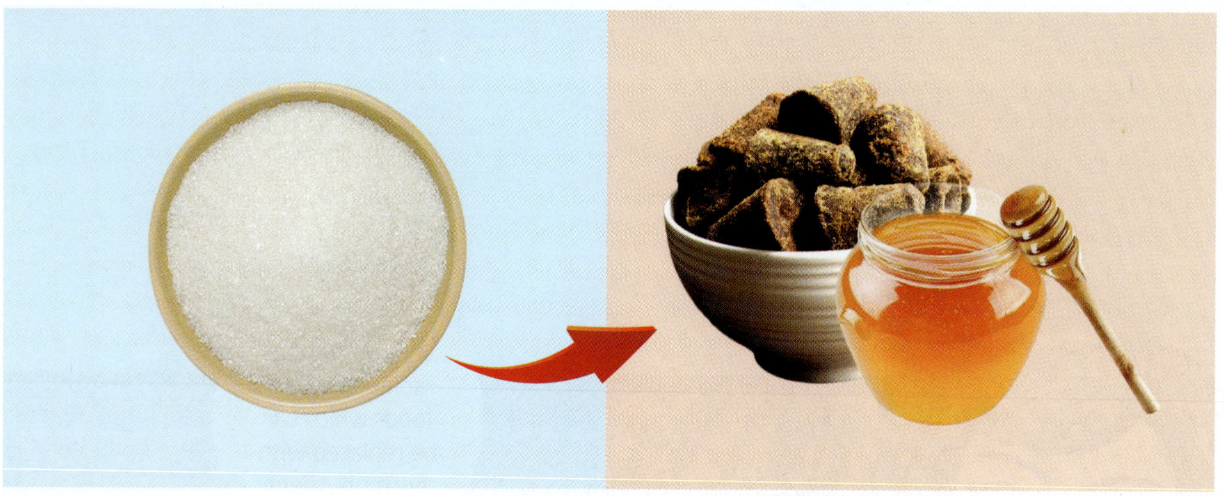

Soft Drink to Buttermilk, Sattu, Home-made Sherbets, Coconut Water.

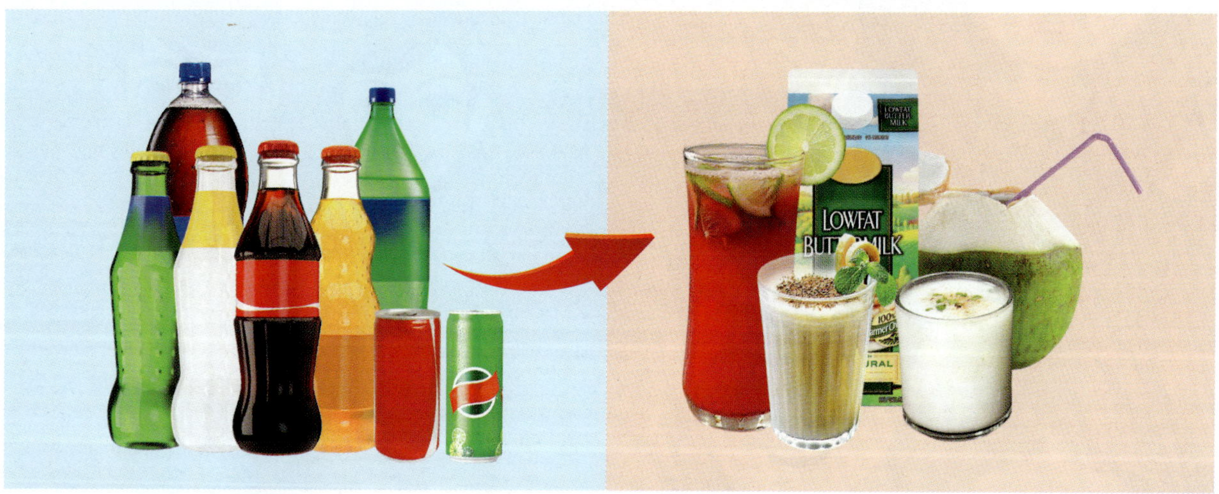

Rice and Wheat to Millets like Jowar, Raagi and Bajra.

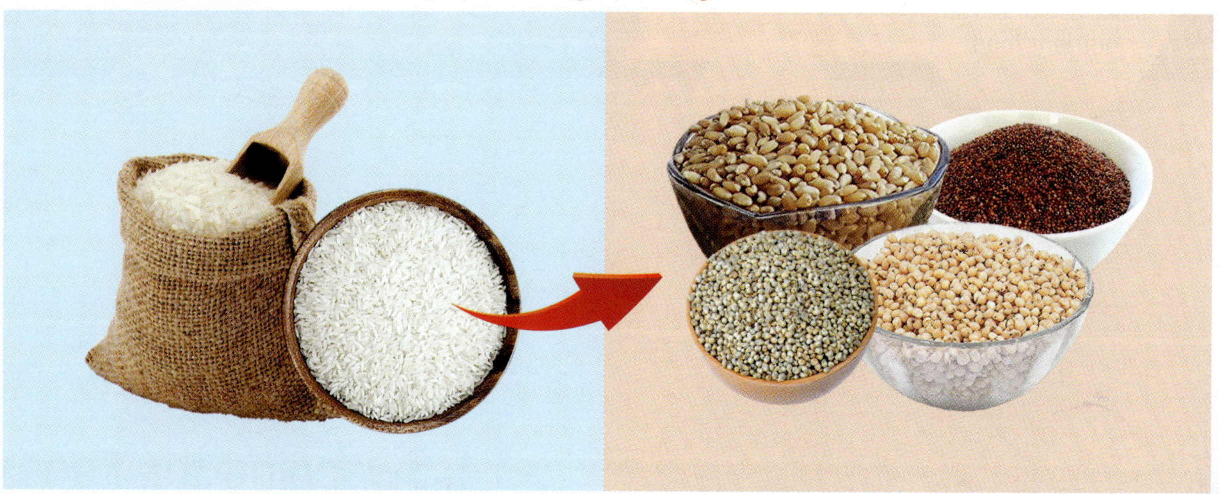

Dal to Sprouts and Pulses.

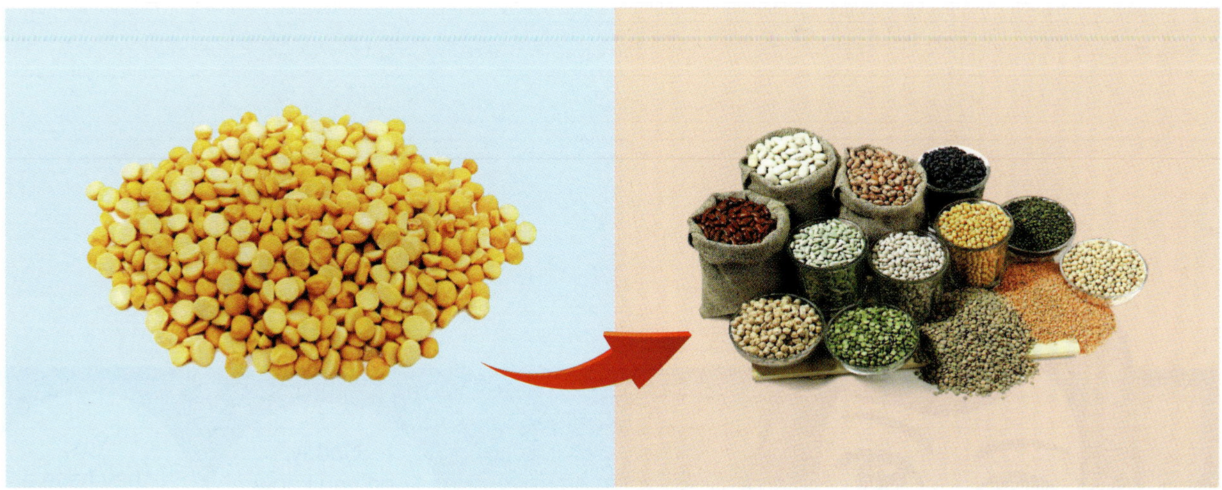

Bad fat to Good fat

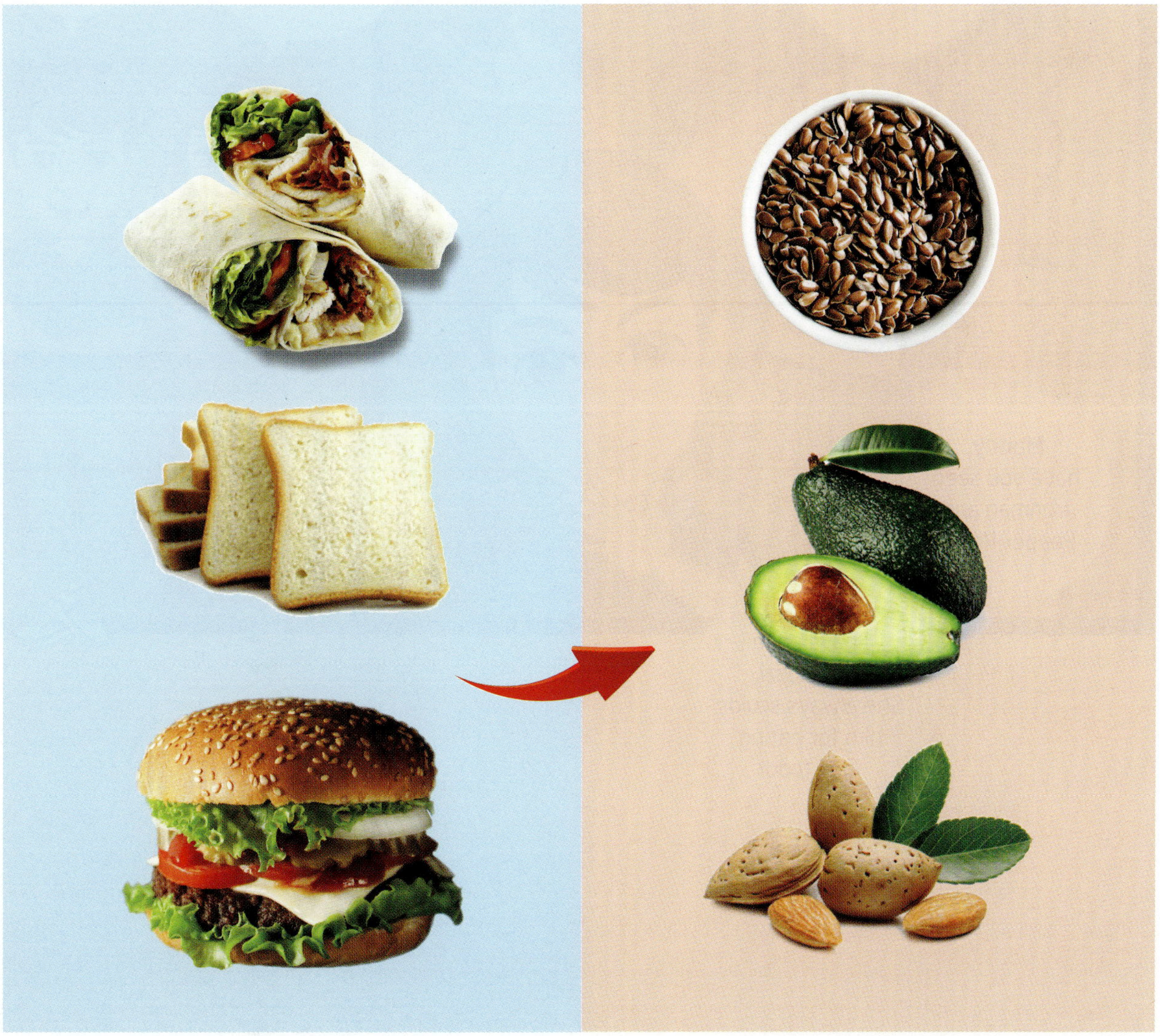

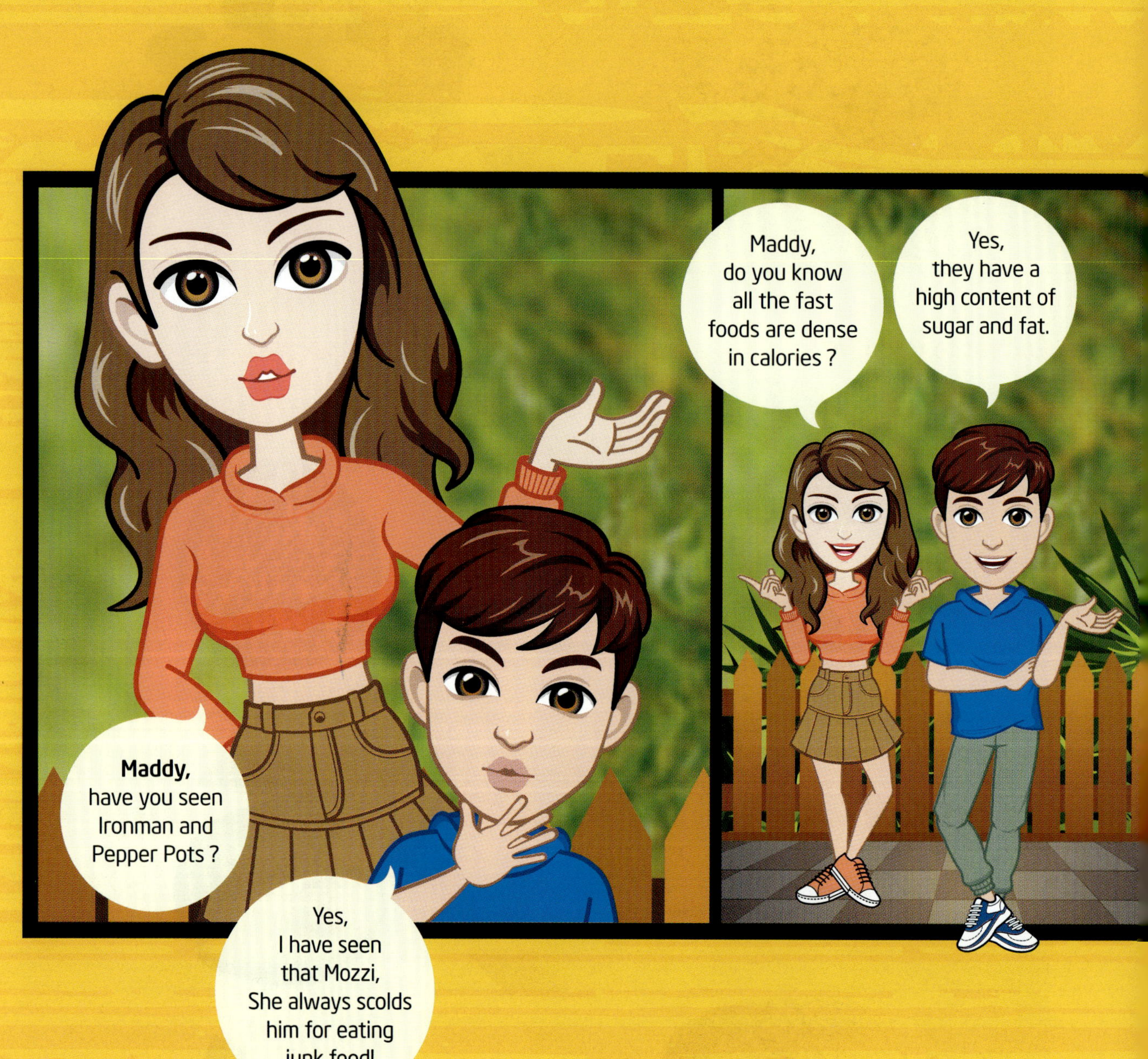

Maddy, have you seen Ironman and Pepper Pots ?
Yes, I have seen that Mozzi, She always scolds him for eating junk food!
Maddy, do you know all the fast foods are dense in calories ?
Yes, they have a high content of sugar and fat.

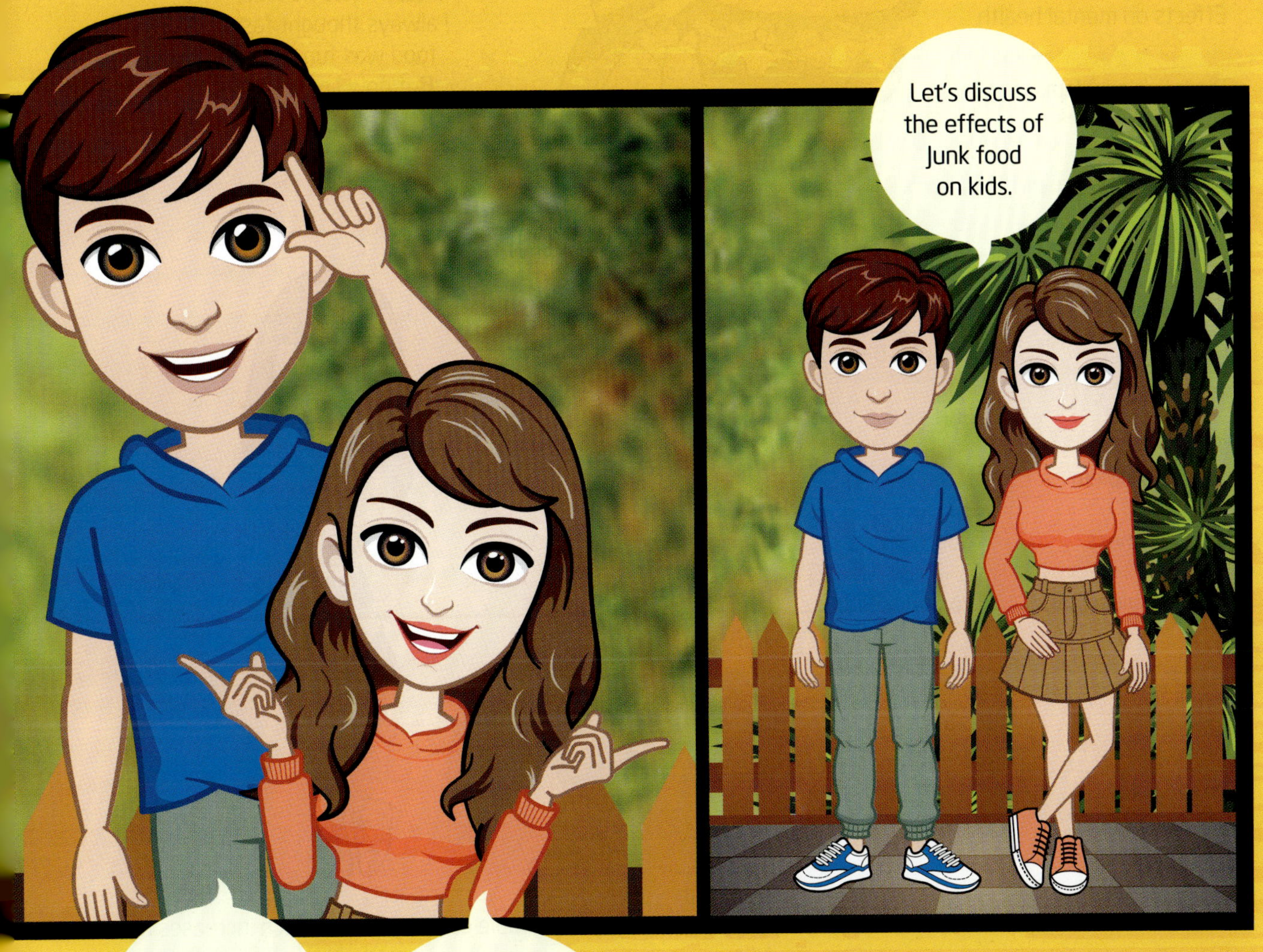

15. Side-Effects of Junk Food

Side-Effects of Junk Food on Kids

Obesity	
Lack of Energy	
Nutrient Deficiency	
Effects on mental health	
Digestive problems	
Constipation	

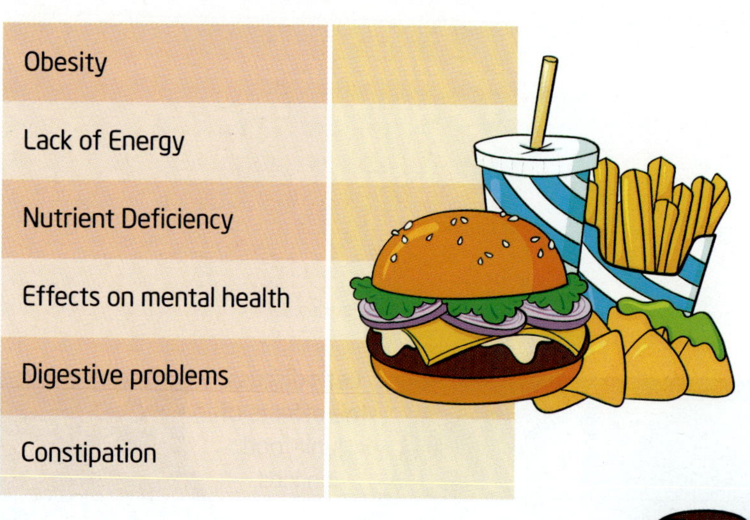

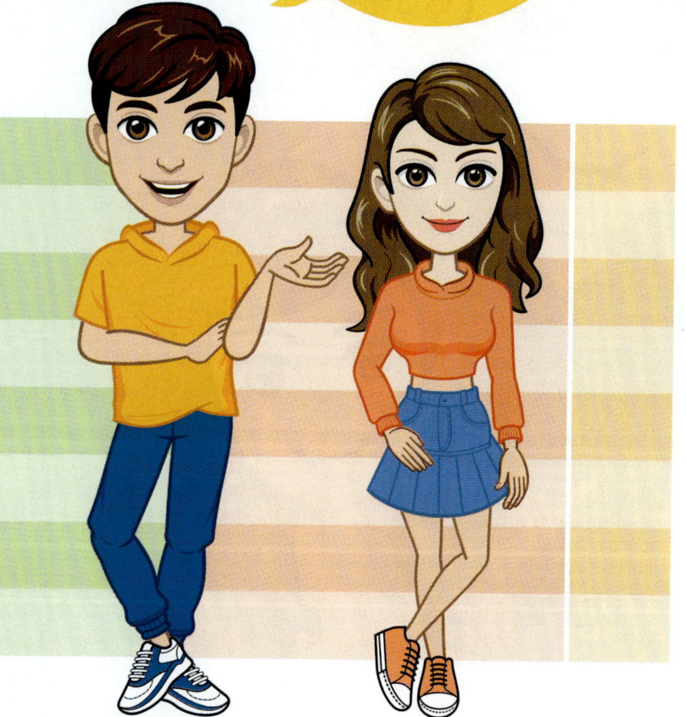

Junk Food VS Healthy Food

Obesity	Healthy BMI
Diabetes	Energetic
Heart problem	Brain Fitness
Sluggishness	Good Memory
High Cholesterol	Positive Mood
Addiction	Overall Health
Illness	Happy Life
Depression	

1. There are many ways in which Junk food may harm your body like simple carbohydrates which increases our insulin resistance.

2. Junk food contains added colours which are harmful for human body and also increase the risk of cancer.

3. The amount of Oil & Fat in Junk food increases the probability of many skin diseases.

4. High sodium affects our Kidneys.

5. We feel drowsy, Soft drinks also numb dopamine.

6. Junk & Fast food do not give any nutrition, instead, they CAUSE liver, Kidney or other syndrome-related human body diseases, loss of memory, depression obesity etc.

"No tablet can completely neutralize the harm done to the individual's health from eating unhealthy. Better ways to reduce your risk of death from heart attack include eating healthy, exercising and maintaining a healthy weight."

Have you ever given a thought what junk food is?

Junk food is not only burger and pizza, junk food is any food which has high calories with fewer nutrients like our shrikhand, samosa and puri.

- Say "NO" to junk food.

- Tracking your food intake – counting your calories and nutrition on day to day basis (Make it a habit of counting calories intake in junk food).

- Whenever craving of junk food arises or any food offered to you, consider the points mentioned earlier. Think about side effects first.

- Discourage your siblings and friends from eating junk food.

- Before listening to your tummy and consuming yummy food, listen to your gut and understand which food plays an important role for you.

What Is the Choice When You Eat Outside ?

We love eating out. The reason behind it is that the food is very tasty. Why is it tasty?

- It is tasty because it has lots of added colors and flavors. It also has more sugar and bad oils like vanspati and Palmolive oil.

- It is not healthy; it has no nutrition.

- We celebrate every good occasion in our life with food; be it a school friend's party, or a birthday treat, our festivals, marriages and so on. We cannot avoid eating outside food. We might feel, we are happy and isn't it our right to enjoy it? But small changes can help us to eat healthier food and avoid junk food.

Let's check out how to do that

- Before going outside drink two glasses of water and eat a fruit or cucumber or tomato.

- If you are going for buffet, then apply half plate rule meaning take what you like most and take in less quantity in your half plate and other half plate add salad and dal.

- If you are going for pizza party, avoid cold drinks and fries. Satisfy yourself with two slices only.

- Drink lots of water which will help you to satisfy your temptation.

- smartly order dish which has good content of vegetables. Ask them for extra vegetables instead of extra cheese. (If you are watching some movies or series of Japan, Korean and China you understand they order veggies and eat less rice or noodles).

We are a smart generation and we should show our intelligence here as well !

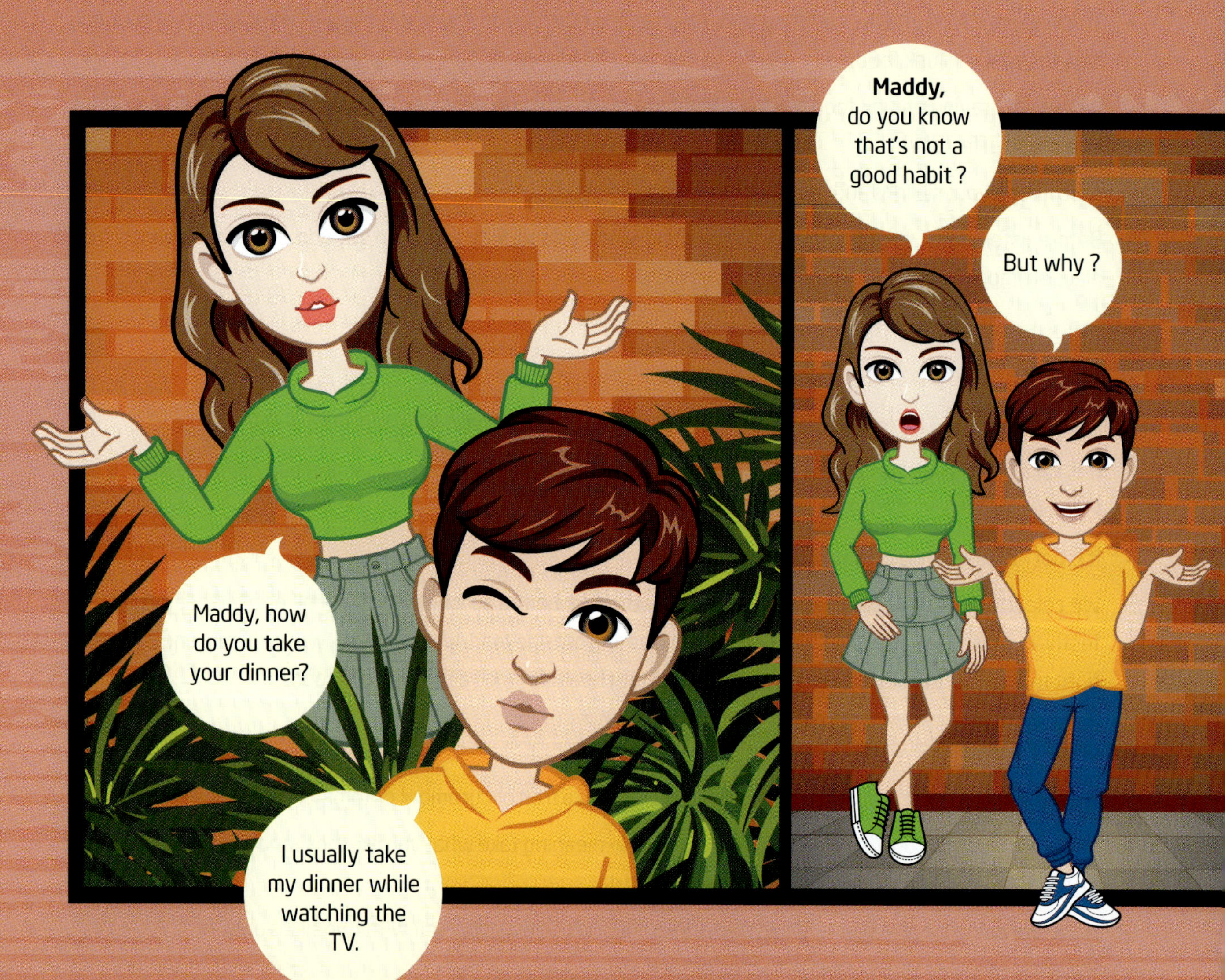

Maddy, how do you take your dinner?
I usually take my dinner while watching the TV.
Maddy, do you know that's not a good habit ?
But why ?

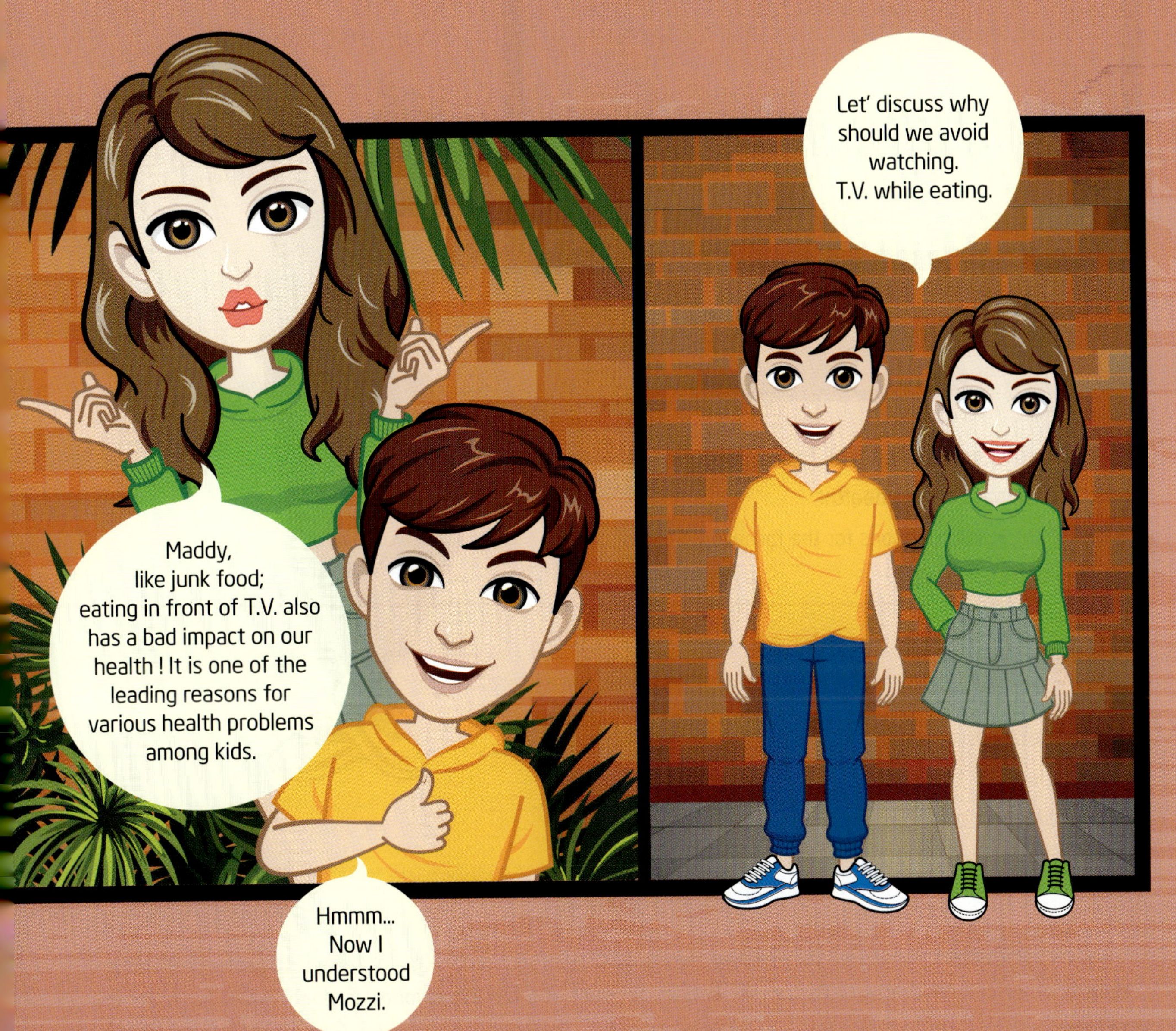

16. Eating in front of T.V.

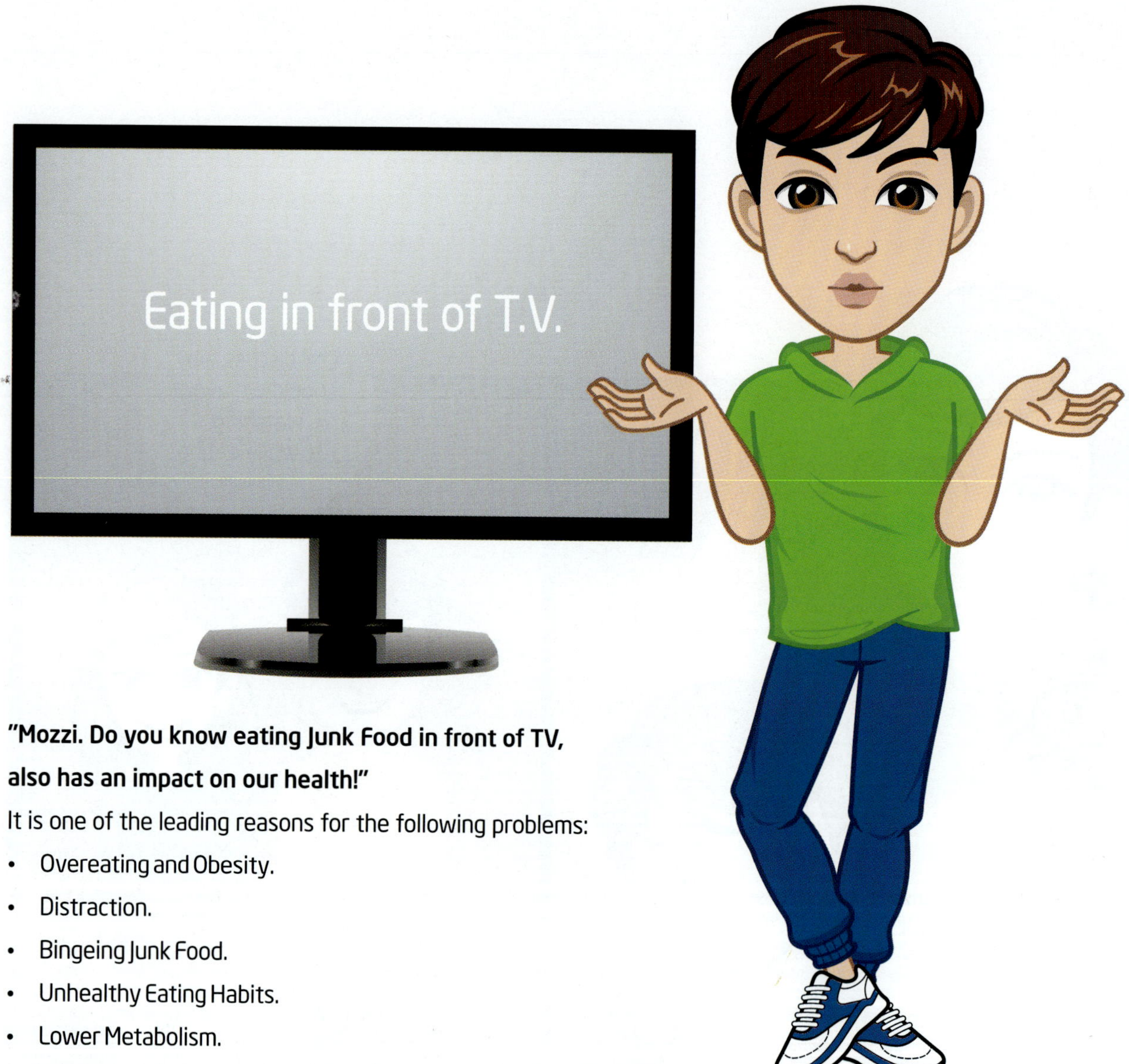

"Mozzi. Do you know eating Junk Food in front of TV, also has an impact on our health!"

It is one of the leading reasons for the following problems:

- Overeating and Obesity.
- Distraction.
- Bingeing Junk Food.
- Unhealthy Eating Habits.
- Lower Metabolism.
- Indigestion.
- No Satisfaction.
- No Family Interaction

Food Fact

Food advertising aimed at children- for example, during kids' TV programs-is 70% for fatty & sugar foods,16%for cereals & other carbohydrates, 10% for milk & dairy product, 4% for fish & meat products & 0% for fruits & vegetables.

Eating whilst watching T.V reduces diet quality. We eat food with high fat content or high sugar content. Fruits and vegetables consumption goes down. We also end up having a high number of sugar sweetened beverages.

Food Fact

When the food commission looked at 385 products targeted at children, only one in ten could be regarded as healthy, while over 75% contained excessively high levels of saturated fat, sugar & salt.

- When we are multitasking, our brain is not so mindful of eating.

- Our brain cannot give signals to our digestive system to inform us that we are full.

- So, while eating food, please only focus on "eating food".

According to a research paper, long time spent on TV viewing, and possibly to a lesser degree, frequent consumption of meals during TV viewing, seem to be associated with generally having unhealthy food preferences and food habits among school-going children.

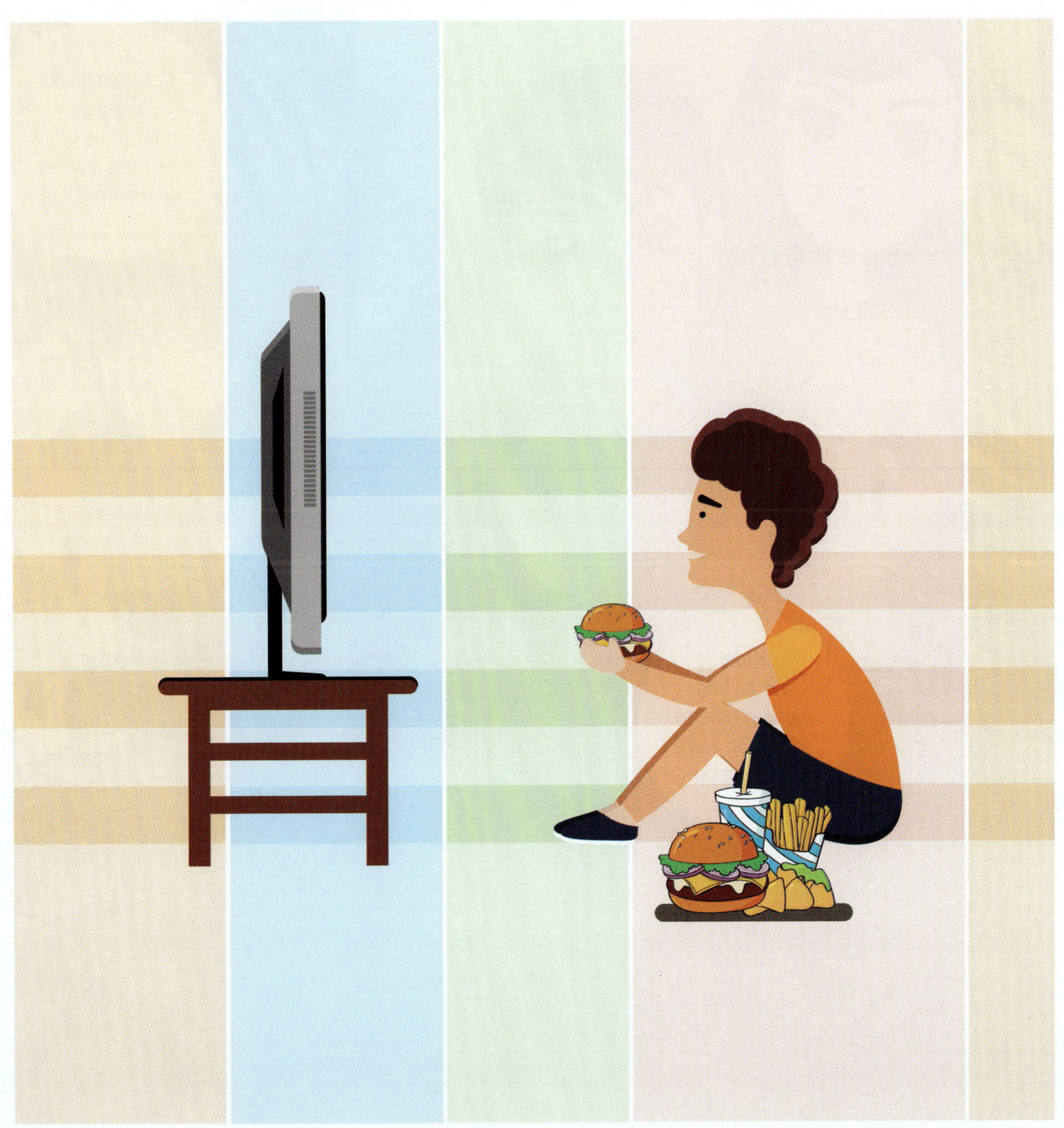

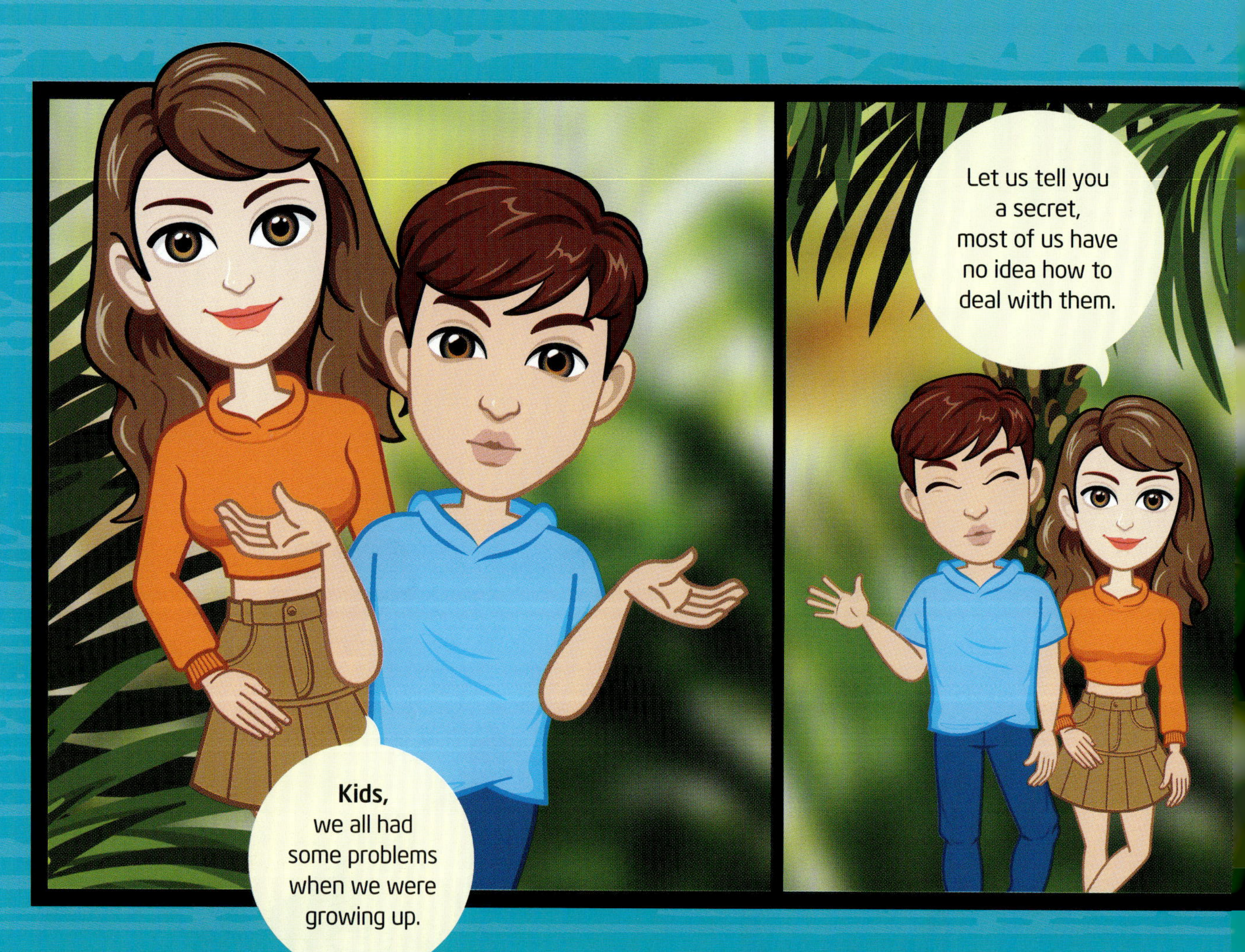

Kids, we all had some problems when we were growing up.
Let us tell you a secret, most of us have no idea how to deal with them.

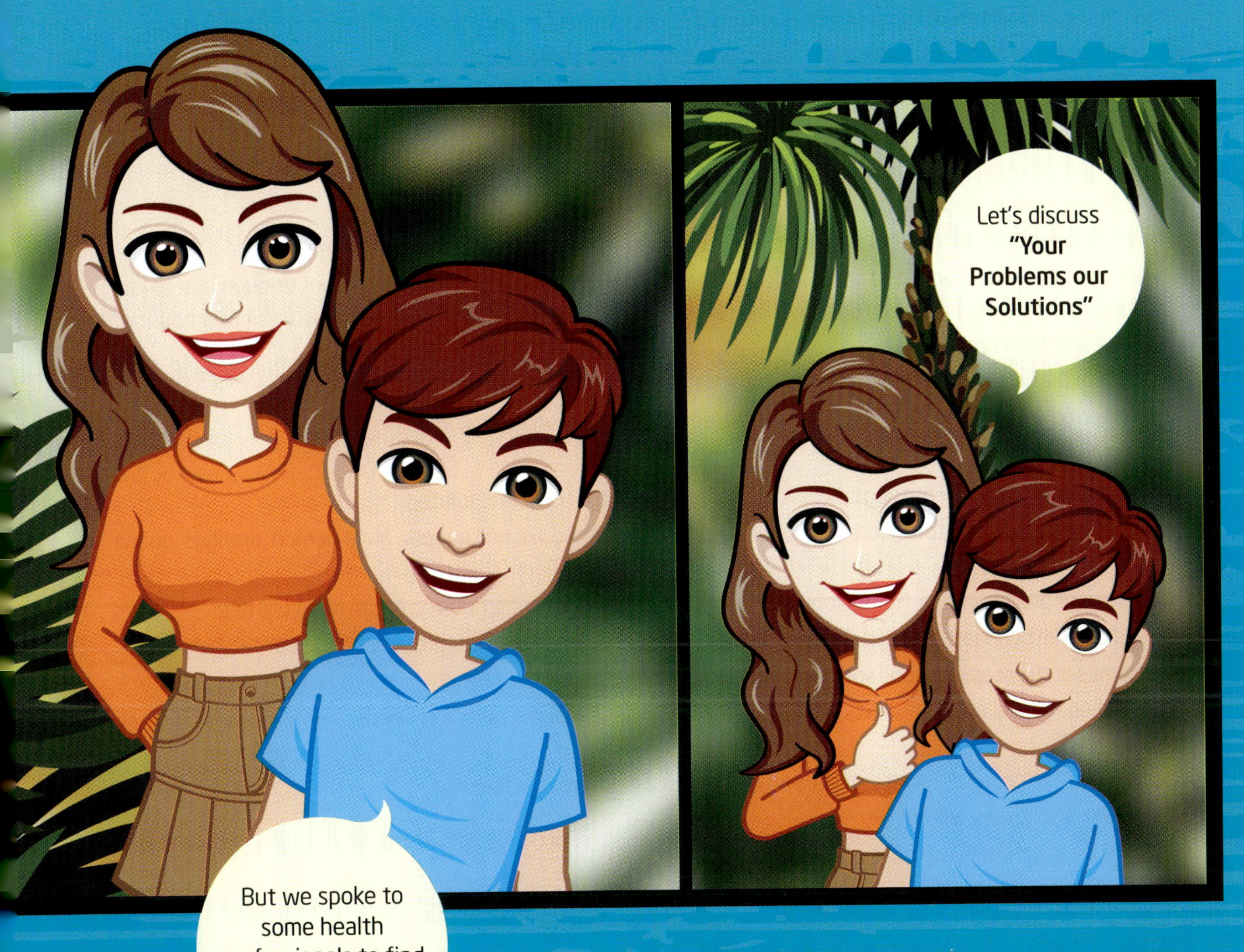

17. Your Problems Our Solutions

Acne

Acne is mainly seen in teenagers and occurs when hair follicles or pores are plugged with oily secretions from skin oil glands. This blockage is known as a white head or black head. But sometimes it develops into a swollen red tender bump.

How to tackle Acne?

- Drink lots of water because water helps to excrete toxins from your body through urine and perspiration.
- Avoid dairy products on trial basis.
- Consult your dietician or a doctor for the right intake of milk and milk products.
- Avoid high sugar as it spikes your insulin level which increases sebum production.
- Increase intake of zinc and selenium. (Refer sources of Zinc and Selenium)
- Eat more vitamin A and C. (Refer sources of vit. A , E, C)
- Eat fiber rich diet so your gut is in good condition.

Anemia

Anemia is a condition when your red blood cells are less.

There are many types of anemia, but iron deficiency and pernicious anemia are the most common ones.

In Iron deficiency anemia, red blood cells (which deliver oxygen throughout the body) are not enough due to low hemoglobin. Hemoglobin is made up of hem = iron and globin = protein. So, when we have insufficient amount of iron, we have low hemoglobin.

Pernicious anemia occurs when your folate and vitamin B 12 is less.

If you are anemic, you will experience tiredness, extreme fatigue, drowsiness and hair loss.

How to tackle Anemia?

- Increase intake of green leafy vegetables especially spinach as it contains folate.
- Vitamin C rich food helps to absorb iron, so eat vitamin C rich food like bell pepper, amla , lemon ,oranges ,guava and strawberries.
- Increase your protein intake. Hemoglobin is made up of proteins, so eggs, poultry, organ meat will help.
- Eat less calcium rich food if you have severe deficiencies because calcium interferes in the absorption of iron.
- All legumes and pulses are good sources of iron and protein.
- Nuts and seeds are good sources of iron. So, add peanuts, almonds, pumpkin seeds, sunflower seeds, black sesame seeds.
- Garden cress is a good source of iron; so, you can have it as a sharbat or kheer.
- Khajur (dates) chutney will help.
- Eat curry leaves chutney with lemon.

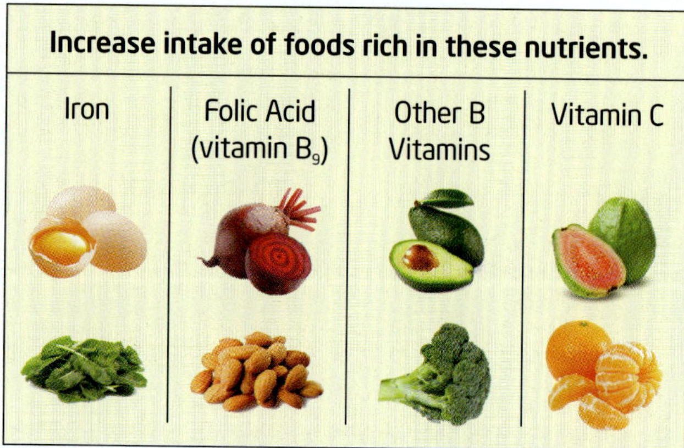

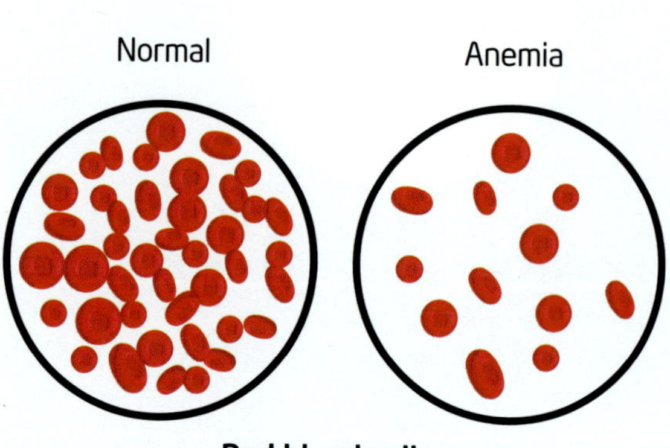

Height

How to increase the height?

- Take a balanced diet which includes vegetables, fruits, whole grains, proteins and dairy products.
- Take more protein in diet.
- Do more stretching exercise.
- Girls need more exercise after the age of 11.5 yrs. and need less fatty and sugary foods.
- Have more calcium, zinc, magnesium and vitamin D for strong and healthy bones which will help to increase your height.
- Good amount of sleep –age 12 to 17 – 9 to 10 hours sleep.
- Yoga also helps to increase height, like "Tadasan".
- Correct your posture.

Obesity

- Child obesity is more dangerous than adult obesity.
- To find out the causes for this you need to examine your blood for serum insulin, TSH (thyroid) so visit your doctor, don't ignore it, it's not a natural process. We need to find out the reasons.
- Please try and understand what increases your fat cells. Mainly there are only two ways to avoide obesity i.e. Exercise and Diet.

Fat Fact

An average man has about 26 billion fat cells, called adipocytes, in his body while a woman has around 35 billion. When people put on weight, the fat cells first actually increase in size, then later multiply.

How to tackle Obesity?

- Drink plenty of water so your hunger pangs are less.
- Do one hour of rigorous exercise.
- Eat lots of high fibre vegetables. Since its absorption is less so it makes you feel satiated.
- Use smart watch or some app to check your calories intake and expenditure.
- Be careful while eating outside. Always use 80/20 stomach equation.
- Take a high protein diet because, it increases your BMR.
- Eat less carbohydrates during meal and take more proteins like 2 katori dal, soya nuggets, paneer, non-vegetarian food, rajma, beans, chole, sprouts, etc.
- Have sattu once a day. It's an Indian high protein drink.
- Keep some handy snacks like roasted peanuts, dry fruits, makhana, murmura (puffed rice).

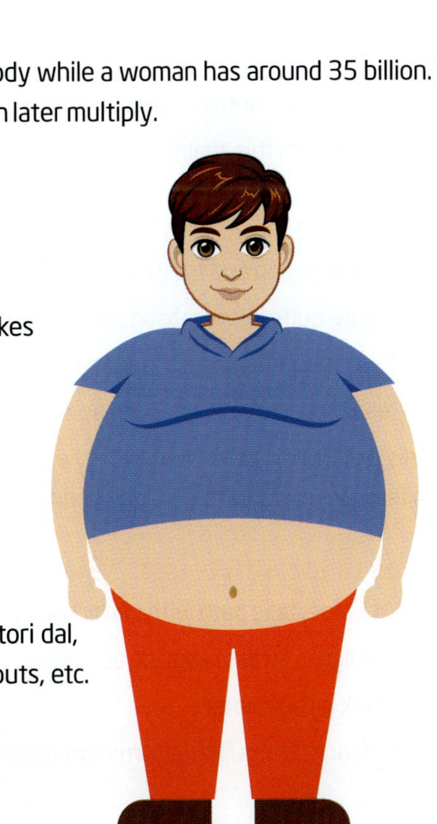

Underweight

Though we have been given age / weight guidelines by doctors, it does not always mean that you are underweight. Only weighing scales are not a measure of your weight.

If you are active and have no health issues, then you are not underweight.

Instead you are healthy.

But if you feel tired, exhausted, then you might be underweight.

How to have a healthy weight?

- Make your digestive system strong. Increase your good bacteria by eating green leafy vegetables, bananas, and curd.
- Drink good amount of water in the form of lassi and sherbet.
- You can add gadii shakkar in your daily water bottle.
- Calculate your protein intake and eat accordingly.
- Eat more carbohydrates like banana, potato, chikoo, mango, sweet potato.
- Keep snacks box with you; eat chikkis and rajgeera ladoo whenever required.

Eczema

It is a common condition affecting children and, usually runs in families having a history of allergies and asthma. It looks like a red, itchy, dry patches over skin especially over the skin creases of hands, wrists, elbows and knees.

It is a chronic condition, but can be controlled with some precautions

How to tackle Eczema?

- Use mild soaps. Take daily but short baths and use lots of moisturizer.
- A ceramide containing moisturizer is a good option, as it helps to repair skin barrier.
- Apart from this, maintain a constant room temperature, wear cotton clothes and avoid scratching any rash.

Excessive Sweating

This is a common and frustrating problem, especially among teens.

There are quite a few reasons for it, but the main causes are:-

A) Excessive function of our body's sweat control system.

B) Response to a stimulus such as medications, anxiety and some neuroendocrine disorders.

This condition can affect the daily activities of the individuals. Excess sweating can occur over palms, feet, face or in few cases, whole body. This condition most of the times requires medical help.

How to tackle Excessive Sweating?

- At home, take bath with water, which has been mixed with alum, twice a day to control the situation.
- Indulge in stress reducing activities.
- Drink lots of water.
- Eat more fruits like watermelon-muskmelon and oranges.

Dandruff

It is a common condition affecting scalps in both children and teens.

It is produced when skin of scalp exfoliates and can be seen as white flaky material in hair and shoulders. Dandruff alone cannot cause any problems, but seborrhea, most common cause of dandruff can cause red, itchy rash over scalp.

Sometimes ears, face, mid chest and mid back can also be affected.

How to handle Dandruff?

- Avoid using hair oil over scalp.
- Do not scratch your head.
- Use good anti dandruff shampoos containing zinc pyrthione, selenium sulfide, ketoconazole at least twice a week.

Greying of Hairs

This problem is increasingly seen in children and teens mainly due to unhealthy lifestyle and unwanted stress they are subjected to when greying of hair occurs in children less than 20 years of age, it is called premature canities.

In children, it is mostly due to common nutritional disorders like protein energy malnutrition and micronutrient deficiencies like iron and zinc.

In teens, excessive crash dieting and overuse of hair cosmetic products, stress and lifestyle changes can cause greying of hairs.

How to handle Greying of Hairs?

- Adequate supplementation of macro and micronutrients can help in turning back the grey hair to black.
- Stop overusage of hair care products.
- Have a healthy diet.
- Avoid stressful situations.

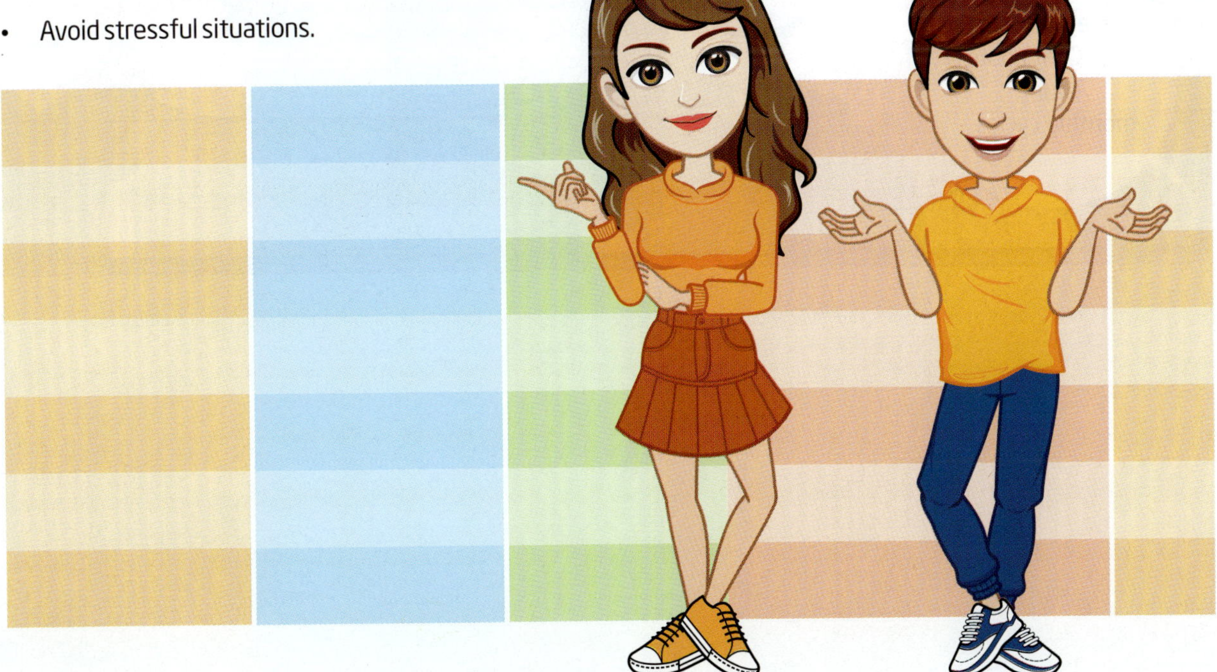

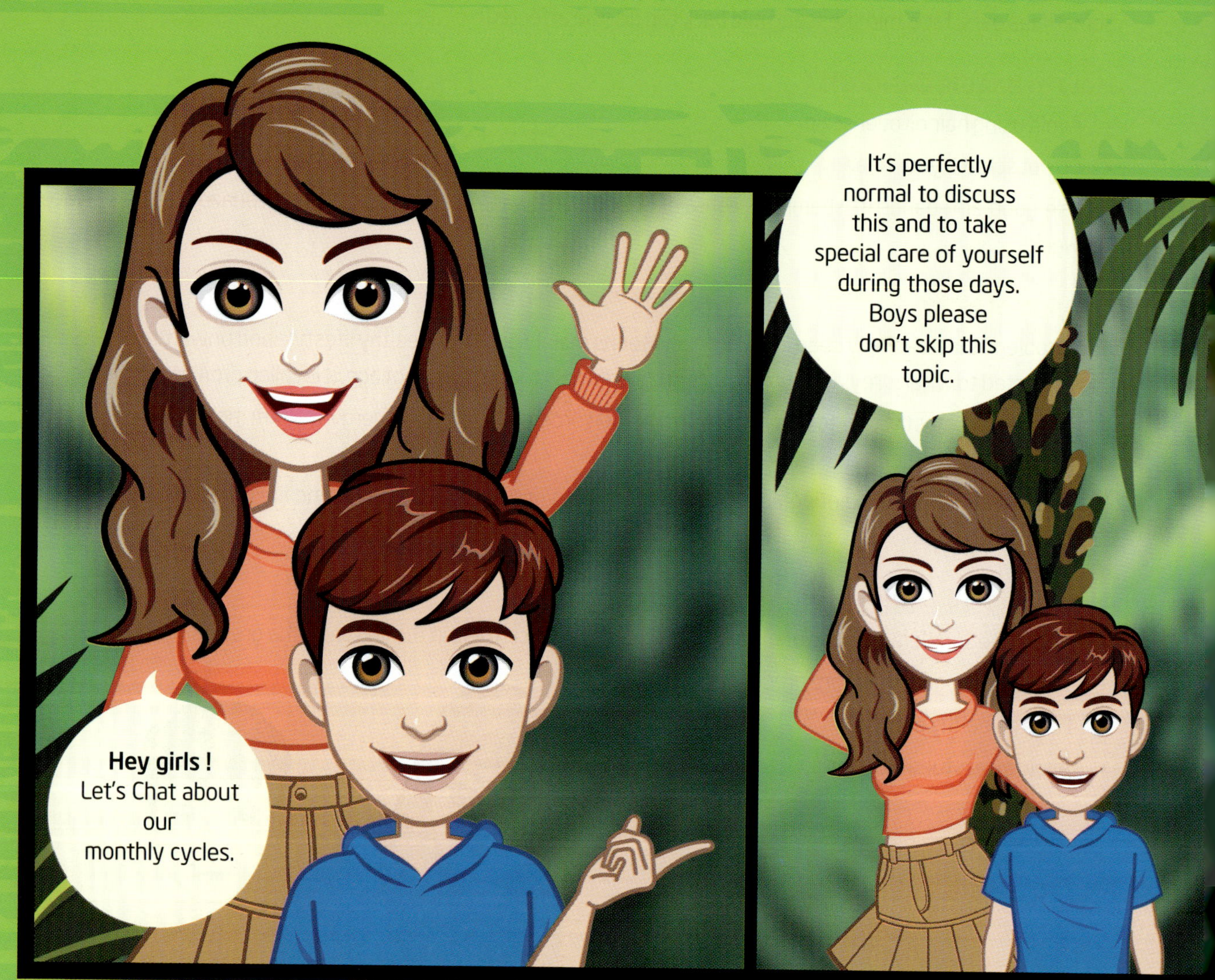

Hey girls !
Let's Chat about our monthly cycles.
It's perfectly normal to discuss this and to take special care of yourself during those days. Boys please don't skip this topic.

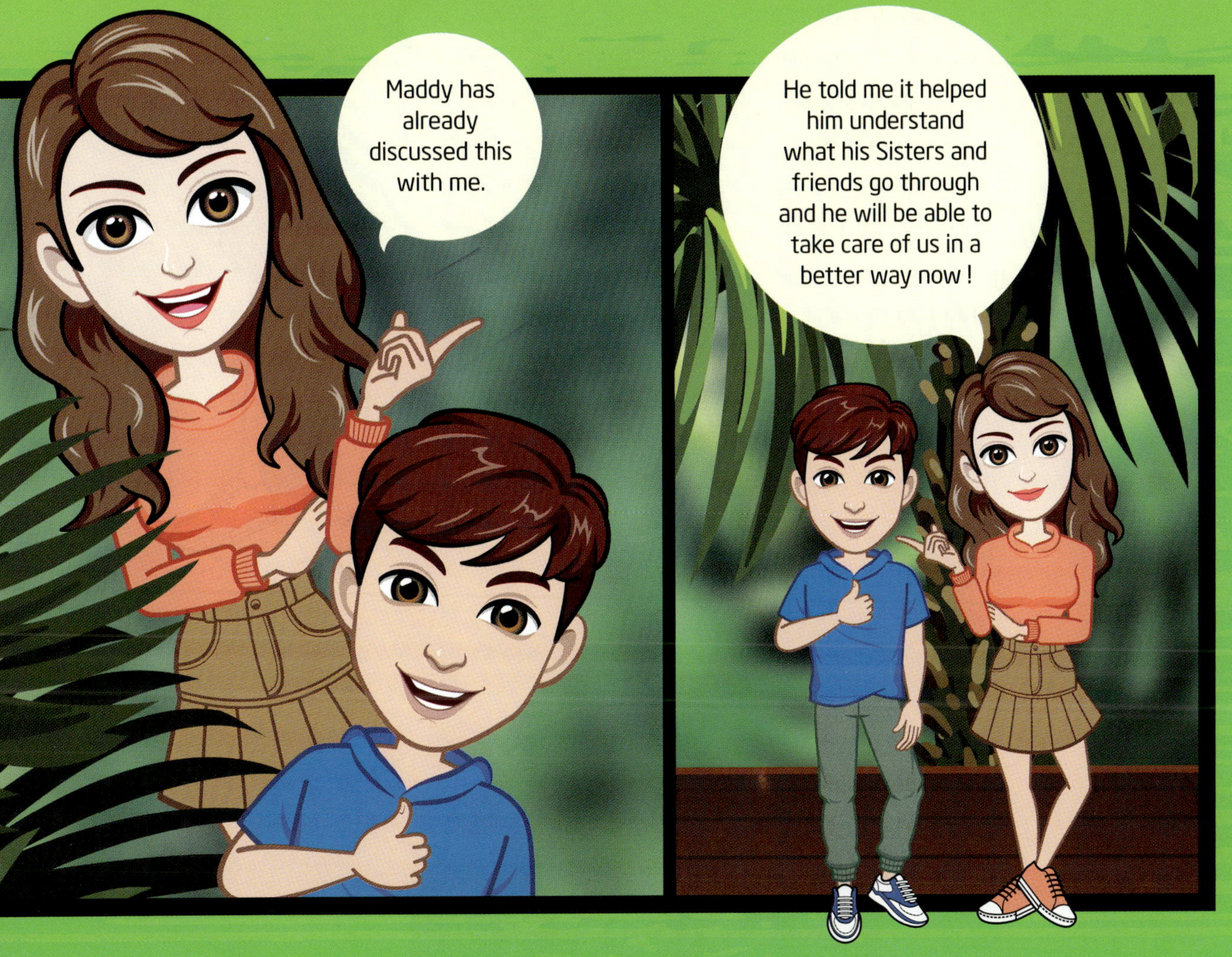

18. Menstrual Cycle

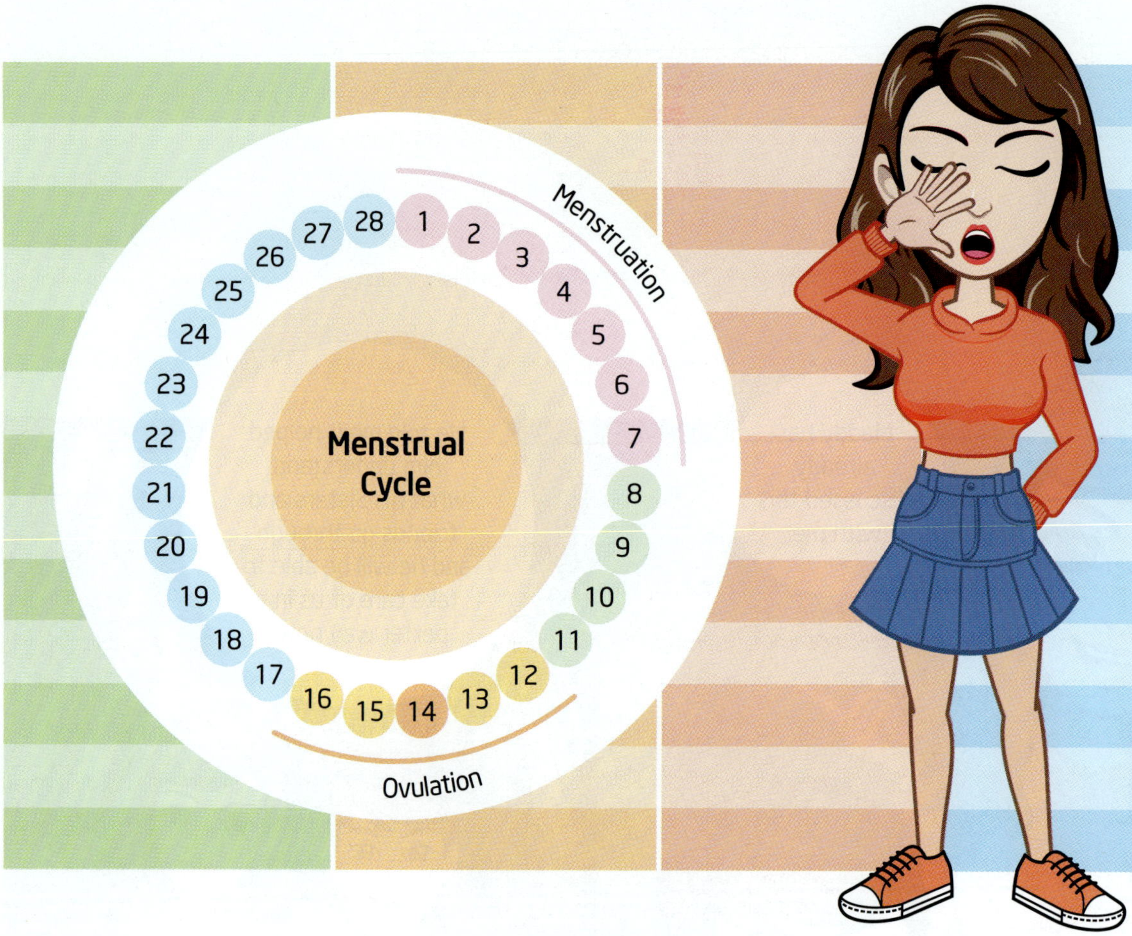

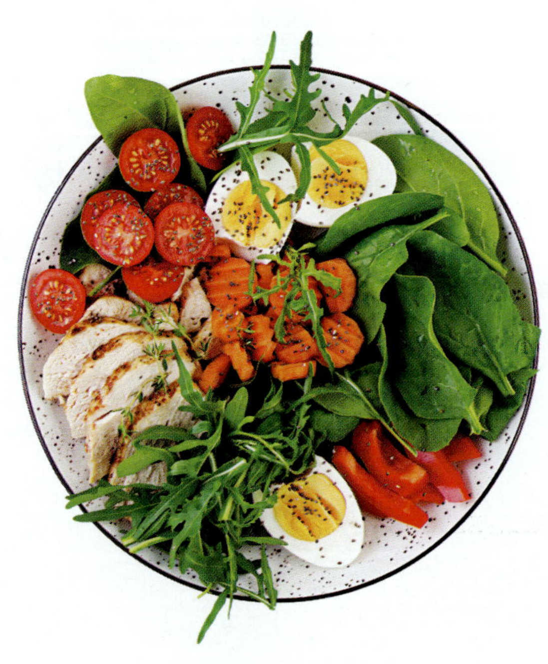

Balanced Diet

What is a menstrual cycle?

- Each month during the years between puberty and menopause, a woman's body goes through a number of changes to get it ready for a possible pregnancy. This series of hormone-driven events is called the menstrual cycle.
- During each menstrual cycle, an egg develops and is released from the ovaries. The lining of the uterus builds up. If a pregnancy doesn't happen, the uterine lining sheds during a menstrual period. Then the cycle starts again.
- A woman's menstrual cycle is divided into four phases:
  a. menstrual phase
  b. follicular phase
  c. ovulation phase
  d. luteal phase
- Once girls start having menstrual cycle, hip: waist ratio as well as weight increases. So, we need to do a combination of exercise = yoga + exercise/ physical exercise + dips (for proper breast development).

Here are few suggestions for healthy menstruation cycle:

- If you have cramps apply heat pads on abdomen
- Avoid soft drinks, sugary, salty and fried foods during periods.
- Drink ginger mint water.
- Increase intake of pyridoxine vitamin – sources- are fish, beef, liver, meats, potatoes, yams and other starchy vegetables, eggs.
- Increase intake of papaya and other water rich foods like watermelon, cucumber.
- Increase intake of fruits and vegetables.
- Fennel seeds, cinnamon, turmeric are good spices in menstruation cycle. You can add in water and have it.
- Walnuts, almonds, flax seeds and pumpkin seeds are good sources of omega 3 fatty acids which are anti-inflammatory.
- Drink lots of water which helps to reduce water retention.
- If you have cramps increase intake of calcium rich food.
- If your periods are irregular do proper exercise after your periods because exercise releases endorphins, Yoga too can help you a lot.

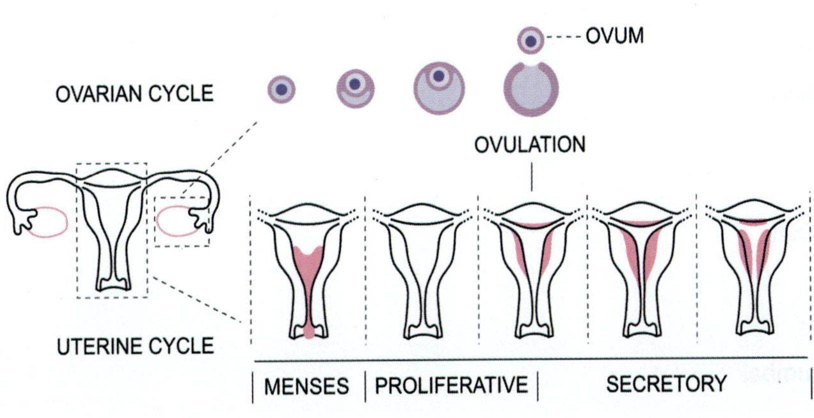

Contact

Meghana Kumare
Dietitian / Nutritionist

M.Sc., PGDD, ISSA (USA), INFS
Clinical & Sports Nutritionist
Corporate Dietitian
Nutrigenomic Counselor
20 years' experience
You can reach us at +91-7774944783 or by email at rawdiets12@gmail.com.
We look forward to working with you!
Follow us on IG - www.instagram.com/meghanakumare

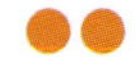

Meghana Kumare is a nutritionist and dietitian running her own center
"Red Apple Wellness Diet Center" in Dubai / Mumbai/ Nagpur / Pune,
Founder of MK FitFoodz, She is lifestyle coach, blogger a motivational
speaker, writer and has innovated many nutritious food products,
some are patented. She has helped many in overcoming weight
management and clinical problem. She has helped sports person in
enhancing life style and performance in their respective sports. She
has conducted many health and wellness workshops. She has given
guest lectures in prestigious institutes such as Tata memorial hospital.
She has conducted seminars and lectures for multiple corporates,
school and NGO's

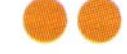

Services

- Weight management
- Sports Nutrition
- Kids Nutrition
- Clinical Nutrition
- Corporate Wellness
- Cancer Diet
- Detox Diet
- Princess Bridal Diet
- Pregnancy Diet
- Women Wellness

Nagpur | Pune | Mumbai

Acknowledgments

Every Book has its own story. Writing a book is surreal process. I am indebted to Mrs. Sapna Sharma, Mr Shripad Aparajeet, Dr. Nikanth Kulsange, Mr. Mukund Patrikar for their inspiration & keen insights, and their ongoing support in bringing my book to life.

Life of book is editor Mrs Dhanshree Sawant, thank you for your narration, Mrs Noopura Kinkar & Mrs. Gauri Dhadharphade for valuable contribution, Mr. Sanjeev Mendhe & Mr. Ashutosh Jangade, who made all the fictional character, lively. Special thanks to Mr. Chitaranjan Yadav for reviewing my book.

There are always some people behind me in my life and their support is infinite such as Mr. Sunil De, Mr. Achal Gandhi, Mrs. Minal Gedam, Dr. Rani Bhutada and Mahie Bhutada my special thanks for their support. My special thanks to Dr. Shashank Bansod for his consultation on hair and skin in this book.

Sara my lovely daughter who used to cook for me whenever I was busy and she had given her views about the book, Being a teenager she understands, what child wants to read and what kid's likes. Her insights are valuable.

My brother late Mr. Komil Kulsange has been a good advisor cum google suggestion box for me. Lastly, I would like to thank my parents, mother in-law for their constant and unconditional support and all others who has supported me in writing this book

Dt. Meghana Kumare

Bibiliograpy

- www.fao.org/nutrition/en/
- www.sciencedirect.com/topics/agricultural-and-biological-sciences/body-composition
- www.pediatrics.aappublications.org/content/pediatrics/102/Supplement_3/507.full.pdf
- www.ncbi.nlm.nih.gov/pmc/articles/PMC4266869/
- www.ncbi.nlm.nih.gov/books/NBK218769/
- www.nutrition.org.uk
- www.cancercenter.com/community/blog/2016/08/natural-vs-refined-sugars-what-is-the-difference
- www.researchgate.net/publication/270000334_Sugar_Intake_Obesity_and_Diabetes_in_India
- www.webmd.com/food-recipes/features/health-effects
- www1.health.gov.au/internet/publications/publishing.nsf/
- www.healthline.com/nutrition/foods/peanuts#vitamins-and-minerals
- www.nutritionaustralia.org/national/frequently-asked-questions/general-nutrition/nuts-and-health
- www.nutritionfacts.org/video/what-about-coconuts-coconut-milk-and-coconut-oil-mcts/
- www.en.wikipedia.org/wiki/Vitamin_A
- www.ncbi.nlm.nih.gov/pubmed/29597234
- www.en.wikipedia.org/wiki/B_vitamins
- www.healthlinkbc.ca/health-topics/ta3912
- www.wholesomebabyfoodguide.com/iron-and-iron-rich-baby-foods-what-iron-rich-foods-can-baby-eat/
- www.fao.org/3/Y2809E/y2809e0j.htm
- www.fao.org/3/Y2809E/y2809e0j.htm
- www.ncbi.nlm.nih.gov/pmc/articles/PMC4337919/
- www.medlineplus.gov/ency/article/002412.htm
- www.msdmanuals.com/en-sg/home/hormonal-and-metabolic-disorders/electrolyte-balance/overview-of-electrolytes
- www.ncbi.nlm.nih.gov/books/NBK201497/
- www.nccih.nih.gov/health/probiotics-what-you-need-to-know
- www.nccih.nih.gov/health/probiotics-what-you-need-to-know
- www.researchgate.net/figure/Amla-fruit-chemical constituents_tbl1_331857453
- Images: www.freepik.com
- BMC PUBLIC HEALTH 2011; 11: 311.
  Published online 2011 May 13. doi: 10.1186/1471-2458-11-311
  PMCID: PMC3112126
  PMID: 21569476

- C. Gopalan, B. V. Rama Sastri, S. C. Balasubramanium, "Nutritive Value Of Indian Foods, National Institute Of Nutrition", (2004).
- Indian Council of Medical Research Nutrient Requirements and Recommended Dietary Allowances for Indians, National Institute of Nutrition, Hyderabad, 2010.
- L. Kathleen Mhan Suivia Escort- stump kravse's food Nutrition and Diet Therapy 10th edition.
- Subhangini Joshi, "Nutrition and Dietetics with Indian Case Studies" 3rd edition.
- Judith Wills "Diet Bible" 2001.

Note

Note

Note